The Doctor Dilei
Public Policy and the Changing Role of Physicians
under Ontario Medicare

The Canadian health care system is undergoing fundamental restructuring that will require important changes in doctors' professional roles. S.E.D. Shortt, a practising physician for two decades, argues that rather than resisting such changes, as has sometimes happened in the past, doctors could make significant contributions to the design and operation of a new system of health care.

The *Doctor Dilemma* provides a timely discussion of policy issues in five key areas of physician-related public policy in Ontario: physician payment schemes, regulation of the number of physicians and their distribution, monitoring of the quality of medical care, the role of physicians in hospitals, and the regulation of new medical technologies. Shortt defines the scope of the problems, clarifies the focus of the debate, identifies the constraints on policy formation, and discusses the policy options available. He accepts the inevitability of substantial change to the health care system and the way practitioners work but believes that if doctors take part in the process such change can ultimately lead to a better system of health care in Ontario. The *Doctor Dilemma* puts the debate into a balanced context and helps pave the way to finding solutions.

S.E.D. SHORTT is director of the Queen's University Health Policy Research Unit and professor in the Departments of Community Health and Epidemiology and Family Medicine.

The Doctor Dilemma

Public Policy and the Changing Role of Physicians under Ontario Medicare

S.E.D. SHORTT

McGill-Queen's University Press
Montreal & Kingston · London · Ithaca

© McGill-Queen's University Press 1999
ISBN 0-7735-1793-6 (cloth)
ISBN 0-7735-1794-4 (paper)

Legal deposit first quarter 1999
Bibliothèque nationale du Québec

Printed in Canada on acid-free paper

McGill-Queen's University Press acknowledges the
financial support of the Government of Canada
through the Book Publishing Industry Development
Program for its activities. We also acknowledge the
support of the Canada Council for the Arts for our
publishing program.

Canadian Cataloguing in Publication Data

Shortt, S.E.D. (Samuel Edward Dole), 1947–
    The doctor dilemma: public policy and the changing
    role of physicians under Ontario medicare
    Includes bibliographical references and index.
    ISBN 0-7735-1793-6 (bound)
    ISBN 0-7735-1794-4 (pbk.)
    1. Physicians – Government policy – Ontario.
    2. Medical policy – Ontario.   I. Title.
    R463.06s56 1998   362.1'72'09713   c98-901192-5

This book was typeset by True to Type in 10.5/13
Baskerville.

Contents

TABLES

Preface

Whether working as a family practitioner or as a teacher of health policy, I have observed that Ontario's physicians are an increasingly unhappy and puzzled lot. On various occasions they seem to see at least three groups as adversaries. First, they see the provincial government as insensitive to their contributions, choosing instead to blame a disproportionate number of health-care woes – which doctors attribute to under-funding, poor planning, and abuse of the system by patients – to physicians. Second, the academic community of health-policy commentators, economists, and epidemiologists offers relentless theoretical critiques but lacks the clinical background to appreciate the realities of medical practice. Third, the public often demands an inappropriate range and volume of services and displays an aggressive consumerism, behind which it raises the ever-present threat of malpractice litigation. Were all this discord not sufficient, there is also clear evidence of internal conflict between specialists and general practitioners over the provincial fee structure and among a variety of medical factions advocating a range of responses towards the provincial government, from complete accommodation to civil disobedience. Small wonder that hard-working and well-motivated physicians are likely to wonder what they did as a profession to deserve a state of chronic confrontation and criticism.

Divided among themselves and perceiving attack from without,

Ontario physicians are, I believe, unwittingly entering the second phase in the evolution of state-sponsored health care. The preliminary period, of approximately two decades, demanded little adjustment by physicians: the only real change was the source of payment for professional services. But in the late 1980s, particularly as provincial governments in Canada faced declining revenues, a new stage in state medicine – "managed health care" – emerged to challenge basic traditions within the medical profession.

The present book is based on my assumption that in Ontario such change is inevitable. I also believe that it does not have to be confrontational and will ultimately lead to a better system of health care. My objective in writing is to describe emerging trends to physicians in the hope that advanced knowledge will enhance their receptivity and participation. I also wish to persuade non-physicians that appropriately credentialled doctors should not be excluded from the design and operation of a new system of health care.

To accomplish these goals I have chosen to discuss five policy issues that I consider central to the physician's role in the gestation of a new health care system for Ontario – paying physicians (chapter 2), the supply of physicians (chapter 3), quality assessment (chapter 4), doctors and hospitals (chapter 5), and physicians and technology (chapter 6). While I concede that other topics might have been included, few informed readers are likely to dispute the importance of the subjects covered. Each chapter defines the scope of the policy problem, specifies factors constraining ready solution, and identifies policy options. These chapters represent policy commentaries rather than formal analysis and are based on a synthesis of the existing literature.

I must at the outset acknowledge my somewhat loose use of terminology. A variety of terms – comprehensive health organizations (CHOS), regionalization, devolution, managed care, integrated health systems – serve below as labels for alternatives to the status quo. The landscape of health policy has changed so dramatically in the last half dozen years that terminology rapidly becomes dated. For the purposes of this book, "devolved" or "regional" authorities simply represent a sub-provincial level of organization determined by geographical or population criteria, for both planning and service delivery. Managed or integrated systems have, among other distinguishing features, a needs-based planning component and, will probably reimburse physicians on something other than a fee-for-service basis.

In completing this manuscript, I have enjoyed the supportive scholarly atmosphere of Queen's University, especially the School of Policy Studies, where I have learned much from both faculty and the students in my policy seminar, and the Department of Family Medicine, where the residents in my seminars are always thought-provoking. I appreciate too the tolerance shown by my practice partners for my arcane interests and all-too-frequent changes in clinical schedules. This manuscript was completed before I joined the Queen's University Health Policy Research Unit; none of my colleagues there is in any way responsible for its deficiencies. My grade-school sons, Mike and Charlie, are also to be commended. Seated at their keyboards they occasionally glance away from the monitor with bemused patience as their techno-peasant father takes fountain pen in hand (a treasured habit now broken by the exigencies of a return to academe). Finally, it has been a continuing pleasure to share a study, an interest in health policy, and a great deal more with my wife, Meri Bukowskyj.

The Doctor Dilemma

Introduction

In the winter of 1996 a physician in Burlington, Ontario, became concerned about the mental status of two individuals. One, a middle-aged male, had apparently developed a monotone style of speech, displayed little facial expression, and engaged in inappropriate behaviour. The presence of a thought disorder or psychosis could not be ruled out. Indeed, stated the physician, the actions of both individuals were possibly dangerous to themselves and were clearly a hazard to others. On that basis he completed paperwork which, under the Mental Health Act, requires police to apprehend the named individuals for the purpose of a compulsory psychiatric evaluation. There was little in this relatively commonplace sequence of events that was likely to excite media attention except for one singular fact: the individuals named by the physician were Ontario's premier, Mike Harris, and its health minister, Jim Wilson.[1]

It would be tempting to dismiss this incident as little more than a perverse attempt at humour by a quixotic physician. But in fact it symbolized a deep resentment and frustration on the part of many Ontario physicians who find their profession buffeted by forces that they did not anticipate and which they poorly understand. This introduction outlines the changing role of physicians, the assumptions underlying medicare at its founding, and the structure of this book.

The contemporary concerns of the medical profession are clearly part of a larger historical process from which the practice of medicine is likely in the near future to emerge in dramatically altered form. From almost unrecognizable roots in the early eighteenth century, physicians by the middle of the twentieth century had evolved to a position of largely unchallenged pre-eminence in the health care systems of developed nations.[2] Indeed, the middle decades of this century in North America may in retrospect look to physicians like a golden age, a time in which organized medicine's claim to diagnostic and therapeutic expertise was recompensed with unfettered professional autonomy and ample financial rewards.[3] Yet it was a transient equipoise. Scholars have pointed to the 1960s as the beginning of the 'decline of medical dominance.' State medical insurance was perhaps the primary factor, but also relevant were challenges from other health professionals, increasing consumer activism, the fragmentation of the profession by gender, speciality, or practice type, and the rise of health bureaucracies, particularly in hospitals.[4] In the United States, the corporate take-over of the health care industry, rather than intrusive government, has been accorded the principal role.[5]

The change in the role of physicians has hardly gone unremarked by the profession. While most Ontario rhetoric is pale by comparison to the vituperation that greeted the introduction of Canada's first state health insurance scheme in Saskatchewan in 1961,[6] the central themes in the health policy debate have remained remarkably constant. For example, the president of the Ontario Medical Association (OMA) for 1985–86, speaking of the government's plan to prohibit extra billing, alleged that its intention was 'the eventual control and subjugation of the profession both economically and medically'.[7]

Some eight years later, little had changed. Faced with the provincial government's 'social contract' retrenchment plan, the OMA charged that the government had 'scooped into its palms the medical profession,' in the process jeopardizing a health care system that, whatever its faults, was 'an enviable model'.[8] Nor were such sentiments confined to the leaders and ideologues of organized medicine. Surveys found that while a majority of Ontario physicians were satisfied with conditions of practice, the rank and file displayed deep anxiety over the changing administrative structure of medicine and their ability to function independently within it.[9]

For once, both the medical hierarchy and its followers were being prescient rather than merely petulant: major structural changes in Ontario's health care system are indeed looming. In his classic study of the medical profession, the American sociologist Eliot Freidson has argued convincingly 'that the truly important and uniform criterion for distinguishing professions from other occupations is the fact of autonomy – a position of legitimate control over work'.[10] Ontario's physicians believe correctly that the autonomy of their profession is currently challenged in a number of key areas – ability to determine the economic conditions of practice; freedom to choose a practice location; the profession's collective right to establish appropriate standards of acceptable practice; its ability to control the institutional workplace; and its freedom to deploy current diagnostic and therapeutic technology without reference to cost. Indeed, the core of medicine's traditional professional identity is threatened by the policy debates in these five critical areas.

For its part, the government of Ontario is equally concerned with these aspects of medical practice. It alleges that fee-for-service payment (see chapter 2) encourages high-volume practice without regard to cost or demonstrable benefits to what is termed "collective health status". It believes that the traditional freedom of physicians to locate where they wish, rather than where they are needed, creates shortages in rural and northern areas and a glut of doctors in Ontario's urban south, which fosters unnecessary use (see chapter 2). It notes that particularly in ambulatory care, both the necessity and efficacy of common diagnostic and therapeutic interventions are unsurveyed and undocumented. The state-financed system is, in effect, paying for a product of unknown quality, a problem that physician-sponsored efforts at quality assurance have done little to resolve (see chapter 3). More than two-thirds of hospital costs, which account for half of the province's health care budget, are generated by physicians, who have, the government claims, little apparent concern with documenting either need or outcome (see chapter 4). Finally, as illustrated by examples ranging from radiographic imaging to the care of acute coronary thrombosis, doctors use technology without reference to expense or efficiency (see chapter 5). These issues have been brought to a head by the almost unprecedented financial constraints facing all levels of Canadian government in the 1990s.

The origin of debates on these matters, however, lies some three decades in the past, in the gestation and early years of Canadian medicare. As is discussed in greater detail in chapter 1, the Ontario government introduced state-funded health insurance in an uncontroversial fashion designed to ensure medical 'business as usual'. The mid-1970s, however, saw the emergence of what was to become a culture of confrontation between physicians and government. It was fuelled initially by government's growing realization that some of the assumptions on which Canadian medicare was founded were simply inaccurate. These convictions, justifiable and even common-sensical in the 1960s, appeared increasingly fragile and naïve a quarter-century later. The struggle to expunge the legacy of these notions is the defining theme of Ontario health reform in the 1990s.

The first of these now-anachronistic beliefs drew on both observed patterns of patients' behaviour in the era antedating state medicine and on the often-impressive record of medical innovation, especially in public health, in the first half of the twentieth century (see Table I). It was assumed that to a publicly funded health system patients would bring only necessary concerns and that physicians would reciprocate by dispensing appropriate scientific care. While the matter is difficult to document, statistics on visits to emergency rooms and family physicians for minor respiratory complaints suggest that some patients trivialize and misuse the system.[11] A growing literature on both inappropriate physician-induced demand for medical services[12] and on marked variation between small areas in the health resources consumed by similar patients[13] suggests that there is no evidence that much of the treatment dispensed by physicians is either consistently scientific or appropriate.

The second credible but ultimately inaccurate assumption informing medicare's founders was also based in part on the seeming success of medicine in the recent past to deal with diseases such as tuberculosis or to devise new therapeutic tools such as penicillin or cortisone. It was assumed that the provision of universal, state-funded care for all Canadians would improve the collective health status of its recipients. But, as a great deal of research suggests, increased expenditures on health care in Ontario and elsewhere cannot be shown necessarily to result in outcomes that enhance population health. To cite the best-known recent example, the

Table 1
Ontario medicare: assumptions and realities

Founding assumptions, c. 1965	Operational realities, c. 1995
Necessary demands are matched with scientific treatment.	Patient misuse; physician-induced demand
	Small-area variations; abuse of technology
Spending more on health care enhances population health.	Unknown correlation between expenditures and outcomes
System requires no management.	Need for managed care with use review and outcome measurement

Black Report, on reviewing the first thirty years of Britain's National Health Service, concluded in 1980 that inequalities in health status had not diminished and in some respects had actually increased.[14]

Here then were two troubling results of medicare unanticipated by the system's founders. The first, broadly conceived, spoke to the problem of use; the second, to measurement of outcomes. Efforts to deal with these two issues became central conceptual pillars in what Americans refer to as 'managed care.'[15] In Canada no notion of management beyond basic financial and administrative activities had concerned the founders of medicare; the system might require supervision, but certainly not active intervention. This hands-off approach was a third incorrect assumption by the system's founders, revision of which became the driving motive in health care reform.

The result of this revision, as considered at greater length below in this chapter, was a scramble by most of the principle participants to articulate their own vision of reform. The College of Family Physicians of Canada, for example, elaborated a thoughtful model for the reform of primary care, which included a blended funding mechanism, use of sophisticated information technology, and an integrated team approach to patient care.[16] The Canadian Medical Association struggled with a number of contentious policy issues, including defining core and comprehensive health services[17] and planning of physician resources.[18] The federal voice was raised by the National Forum on Health in its consideration of many matters, including the correct mix between public and private financing of health care.[19] The Ontario government, echoing moves undertaken in provinces such as Saskatchewan and New Brunswick, created the Health Services Restructuring Commission to rationalize the hospital sector.[20] Set against a background of mounting financial exigency, each of these groups, public or private, contributed to the growing awareness of inevitable change that has defined Canadian health care in the 1990s.

The following chapters, after a fuller description (chapter 1) of the main themes in current health reforms, focus on five specific issues (or policy variables) that relate to physicians – adjusting payment mechanisms (chapter 2); regulating the supply and distribution of doctors (chapter 3); assuring the quality of ambulatory medical practice (chapter 4); revising the role of physicians in hospitals (chapter 5); and creating a rational approach to the deployment of medical technology (chapter 6). Each issue chapter defines and traces the evolution of the problem, documents current policies and constraints on future policy-making, and outlines policy options, while offering suggestions for the preferred alternative. The conclusion brings together policy choices in frameworks based on identified health goals and evaluative criteria and on the five issues analysed in chapters 2–6, and briefly discusses the process of implementation.

1 Context: Reform since 1985

The system of medicare created for Canada in 1966 has enjoyed unquestionable success. On conventional measurements such as life expectancy and perinatal mortality rates, Canada ranks close to the top among developed nations. When compared on more specific grounds with its traditional rival and neighbour, the United States, Canada's publicly financed, universal-coverage system frequently produces roughly comparable outcomes, more equitably distributed. Consider the example of cardiovascular disease. The treatment of myocardial infarction in Canada has been shown to rely markedly less than the United States on coronary care units and invasive procedures, yet both mortality rates and re-infarction rates are largely similar.[1] The presence of chest discomfort and limitation of function one year after infarction are greater in Canadian patients.[2] Seniors in both countries have been shown to have similar access to treatment for cardiovascular disease, except for coronary artery bypass,[3] where the higher American rate appears to favour upper-income patients.[4] There is, in short, no evidence of a marked superiority for the American approach to cardiovascular health care.

Other types of medical intervention also fail to show a significant Canadian deficiency. For example, after reviewing eleven common surgical procedures, a study of Manitoba and New England concluded that low- and moderate-risk procedures fared better in Canada, in contrast to two high-risk procedures which showed better results in the United States.[5] Similarly, while patients in Ontario receiving knee replacements waited longer than their American counterparts, post-operative satisfaction was comparable.[6] While American hospital patients receive substantially more diagnostic testing than do Canadians, much of this difference is attributable to expensive imaging procedures in the elderly,[7] and the benefits of these interventions are unknown. If psychiatric treatment is received by a greater proportion of the population in the United States, the match between needs and services appears more appropriate in Ontario.[8] Finally, American health expenditures include administrative costs, which are at least twice as high per person as those in Canada.[9] While acknowledging the pitfalls of cross-border comparisons, it seems fair to conclude that Canada's health care system, even when measured against its affluent neighbour's, fares very well indeed.

Consumer's enthusiasm for the health care system in Canada has been chronically high,[10] and only recently, in the wake of significant funding cuts and restructuring, have there been signs that the public perceives a decline in overall quality of care.[11] Though physicians find much to criticize within the system,[12] a majority of Ontario's practitioners have been found to be content with the circumstances in which they practise,[13] and Canadian doctors in general are marginally more positive in their attitudes than their more affluent American counterparts.[14] Over the first two decades of its functioning, it would seem safe to conclude, Canadian medicare performed well and generally garnered support from patients and providers in return.

Beginning in the early to mid-1980s, a sinister concern intruded on the optimism of both politicians and health bureaucrats in Ontario. It focused on money and had at least three distinct components. First, despite tight global budget control on hospitals and minimal fee increases for physicians, during the 1980s the annual growth rate in the Ministry of Health's expenditures was over 11 per cent. Second, under the federal Established Programs Financing legislation of 1977, Ottawa's contribution to Ontario health care declined precipitously. In 1979–80, Ottawa contributed 52 per cent of funding for education and health, while by 1991–92 this figure had fallen to 31 per cent.[15] Third, the Ontario government appeared unable to realize new sources of taxation revenue – first, because in 1989 the country entered a costly recession, and second, a "tax wall" seemed to have been reached.[16] The result was a quickly rising deficit and a descending provincial credit rating. The combination of growing costs, greatly diminished resources, and a seemingly inexorable increase in service provision had by the early 1990s created a nighmare in health policy.

Nothing concentrates the political and bureaucratic mind like financial exigency. Now the credible accomplishments of medicare were seen to have come at a price. Female life expectancy, for example, placed Canada second in the world only to France. But equally, in terms of total health expenditure as a percentage of gross domestic product (GDP), Canada was exceeded only by the United States. The case of infant mortality was even more disconcerting, for Canada's record was third, behind far more parsimonious Sweden and Finland.[17] Attention was now firmly focused not on what medicare could reasonably claim to have accomplished but on the fact that Canada's system was the second most expensive in the world. Even more important, superior results from nations with less costly systems confirmed the belief, clearly articulated in Canada at least since the Lalonde Report of 1974, that the general population's health depended to a significant degree on factors entirely beyond the formal health care system.

Concerns about the relationship between cost of health care and the determinants of general health had not gone unnoticed by the small Canadian health policy community. Yet these individuals, during the 1970s, appeared to command an uncertain audience and to exert a minimal influence on policy.[18] During the following decade, however, there were indications in Ontario that government was prepared to adopt new ways of dealing with the broader policy community and its networks in an effort to limit the growing instability of the health care system. The medical profession was pushed aside from a central advisory role in policy formation, with its power assumed instead by the provincial bureaucracy.[19] Equally symptomatic of this new approach was a succession of prestigious commissions, including the Ontario Health Review Panel (1987), the Panel on Health Goals for Ontario (1987), the Premier's

Council on Health Strategy, and the Task Force on the Use and Provision of Medical Services. Specific review bodies examined prescription drugs, the Public Hospitals Act, health promotion, midwifery, and regulation of the health professions.[20] Nor was Ontario unique in this search for better ways to deliver health care. From the mid-1980s on, six other provinces established commissions to examine the health care system, and all subsequently published detailed blueprints for reform.[21] In so doing, each province was engaging in a process of restructuring common to most industrialized democracies over the last dozen years.[22]

From the review process in Ontario in the late 1980s a number of themes emerged, which in aggregate marked the public response to the need for reform and innovation. Some voices for reform supported notions such as user fees and privatization or the overt rationing of services, which would if adopted transform the current system. Most proposals, however, were designed to modify the current system so as to retain the established principles of medicare. Chief among the major themes were these five – review of use, quality assurance, measurement of outcomes, needs-based planning, and community-generated planning and delivery of services – consideration of which constitutes the balance of the present chapter and provides a context for considering changes specific to physicians discussed in chapters 2–6.

First, the deployment of health care resources has been largely unexamined in Canada. Increasingly, however, governments and managers are concerned with "utilization review," which compares performance to accepted standards of appropriate care and seeks methods to rectify identified problems. This process has been most conspicuous in the hospital sector and relies heavily on American experience. In 1966 the US Congress legislated a requirement of retrospective review – review after patients leave the hospital – for all institutions participating in Medicare and Medicaid. The yardstick initially used – length of stay – was clearly inadequate and was replaced in the mid-1970s by diagnostic-related groups (DRGs), which grouped conditions requiring similar lengths of stay and incorporated a severity weighting. In 1983 the US government introduced prospective payment, based on costs of the DRG into which the patient fell, rather than the actual costs of individual cases. Suddenly it became crucial for hospitals to know precisely how resources were deployed in all cases so as to ensure that the prospective payment received would cover actual costs incurred. The result was a sudden proliferation of sophisticated monitoring systems such as appropriateness evaluation protocol (AEP); intensity of service, severity of illness, and discharge screens (ISD-A); and standardized medreview instrument (SMI).[23] While evaluation of specific systems has often been equivocal, an extensive literature survey concluded in 1990 that use review had reduced American hospital expenditures by 14 per cent.[24]

Surveillance of use in Canada has been, in comparison, relatively underdeveloped. Hospital costs have not risen as quickly in Canada, suggesting lesser urgency, while the system of funding by annual global operating budgets, in contrast to prospective payment by individual case, has provided no incentives to collect or lower patient-level costs. There may have been greater difficulty in modifying provider's behaviour in Canada than in American proprietary institutions. Finally, the major trigger for Canadian reviews appears to have been not cost control but institutional overcrowding. None the less, according to a 1990 survey of 123 institutions, 80 per cent of Canadian hospitals deploy some use review. Half of these are retrospective only, while the remainder are concurrent – assessing resource use while the patient is in hospital – or a combination of methods. Most administrators stated that improved bed use rather than lower cost was the primary incentive, found medical staff largely supportive of these endeavours, but were unsure as to the precise outcome of these efforts.[25]

A fully developed utilization program for hospitals should incorporate at least four key elements.[26] First, systems such as AEP, ISD-A, and SMI would be used concurrently to assess bed use. Second, strategies would be created to reduce inappropriate admissions, estimated in Canada by several studies to account for between 24 and 60 per cent of adult patients and between 29 and 67 per cent of paediatric patients.[27] Among such strategies are pre-admission screening and testing, mandatory second opinions for surgery, pre-operative patient education, "do-not-transfer" orders on nursing- home residents, and emergency-department quick-response teams. Third, strategies are necessary to reduce length of stay. These include early-discharge planning, expected-date-of-discharge programs, short-stay units, and admission and discharge holding areas. Finally, there must be incentives to encourage physi-

cians to use resources appropriately. These include case management guidelines, education, feedback by peers, and economic
grand rounds or colloquia to enhance cost awareness.

Can such initiatives actually improve the use of health resources?
The example of a program undertaken by the (BC) Greater Victoria Hospital Society is encouraging. In 1985 it began to develop a
case-mix information system, and two years later it had the capacity to identify differences among physicians in case load, severity of
patients' illnesses, resources used for diagnosis, and treatment
results. These data were subsequently coupled with physician-generated clinical criteria to produce performance 'benchmarks'.[28]
An early appraisal in 1990 concluded that the system had significantly reduced numbers of patient days and admissions for less
severe illness. It, along with several other factors, had reduced the
number of patients awaiting placement and increased the proportion of surgery done on an out-patient basis.[29] It seems reasonable
to conclude that utilization review may significantly improve Canadian health-care management.

Closely linked to concerns about use is a second major theme in
health care – quality assurance. This topic is discussed as it applies
to ambulatory care at greater length below in chapter 5, but a brief
summary seems in order here. Quality care must be shown to be
appropriate, in that it is neither neglectful nor harmful; that it is
effective, achieving its therapeutic purpose with no ill effects;[30] and
efficient, in that it deploys the fewest resources necessary to achieve
its purpose. Traditionally quality assessment employs both implicit
and explicit criteria to evaluate the triad of process, structure, and
outcome of care, with outcome including disability, disease, death,
discomfort, and dissatisfaction.[31] This process of assessment provides the groundwork for quality assurance, in which identified
deficiencies are rectified.

In the past, the quality of medical care was simply assumed to be
high, largely on the basis of the credentials of both the physicians
and the institutions providing the care. But this inference is no
longer adequate. Those who pay for care – in Canada, the provincial governments – demand overt evidence that quality is received
in return for payment. Consumers are increasingly aware of their
right to demand proof that their care is of appropriate quality and,
when it is found deficient, are increasingly likely to enter litigation.[32] Finally, research suggests that quality is often lacking in

medical care. Audit-based studies have shown that physicians frequently deviate from consensus-derived standards of practice,[33]
while a voluminous literature on small-area variations suggests that
physicians themselves are puzzled as to what constitutes the best
approach to many common clinical conditions.[34]

The result of such concerns has been a demand for greater evidence of quality from all levels of the system. The traditional
approach of self-regulating health professions in Canada to quality
assurance – often referred to as the "bad apple" approach – is
increasingly seen as inadequate in its emphasis on simple audit to
identify the overtly incompetent.[35] Hospital boards have the
authority to devise and implement quality-assurance programs,
though American experience suggests that they will not find ready
support among physicians.[36] However, the report of the committee
charged in 1992 with reviewing Ontario's Public Hospitals Act
devoted an entire chapter and a large number of recommendations to legislation of quality-assurance programs in all public
institutions.[37] Quality-assessment and -assurance programs, in
summary, will play an expanding role in Ontario. The remaining debates concern only the specific methods and speed of
implementation.

The third and related major trend in health care management,
concerns outcome measurement. Clinical trials of various therapies are usually conducted in ideal circumstances, frequently in tertiary-care academic health centres, and are said to document the
'efficacy' of a therapy. 'Effectiveness' refers to how a treatment per-
forms in the real world, where randomized, double-blind, controlled trials are generally not possible. Instead, researchers
attempt to understand how variations in outcomes are influenced
by differences in the process or structure of care.[38] As in many
other forms of evaluative research of health care, the United States
led the way during the 1980s through projects such as the Medical
Outcomes Study[39] and the investigation by the Agency for Health
Care Policy and Research of the six disorders that account for over
half of American in-patient surgery.[40]

Various outcomes have their own implications for health policy
and their own techniques for assessment. Death, for example, can
serve as an endpoint to identify hospitals whose overall or disease-
specific mortality rates are greater than expected after one takes
into account demographics and case mix. General levels of health

consequent on specific interventions can be measured by instruments such as the sickness impact profile and the Nottingham health profile. Interviews or surveys can assess patients' satisfaction with treatment. While it is unclear whether it is related to objective health benefits, high satisfaction is itself seen as a desirable product. Finally, there are a number of instruments such as the arthritis impact measurement scale that measure disease-specific outcomes.[41] Techniques are available to assess with reasonable accuracy the results of many forms of medical care.

Determining the consequences of medical intervention is obviously central both to evaluating quality of care and to judging the appropriateness of use patterns. But perhaps more significant, documenting results is the essential first step in calculating the economic impact of treatments. Cost-effectiveness ratios measure treatment results in direct clinical units such as years of life gained or deaths avoided. Cost-utility ratios are calculated in units that consider measures of quality, such as quality-adjusted life-years. Cost-benefit ratios attempt to translate clinical outcomes into dollar values.[42] It is information such as these studies provide that ultimately allows a system to make informed judgments about the relative benefits of allocating scarce clinical resources.

The issue of resource allocation points to a fourth trend in the evolution of Ontario's health care – needs-based planning. In the past, allocation has been determined largely by historical patterns of use and the distribution of both institutions and providers. This traditional framework fails to consider the equity of resource distribution either in a horizontal sense (equal needs receive equal resources) or a vertical sense (unequal needs receive unequal resources). This problem can be solved by distributing resources on the basis of relative need – a process that is independent of past patterns of use, is compatible with any predetermined level of expenditure, and maximizes efficiency by maximizing the expected improvement in health status from a given expenditure.[43]

The central problem for this method is finding a useful measure of need. Health care professionals can make detailed studies of the services required to improve the health status of areas or groups. Case registries, such as those that record cancer statistics, could be provided for all relevant conditions. Population-based surveys might ask citizens to identify their health problems and resource needs. Each of these methods is costly and subject to significant reporting errors, suggesting that indirect indicators would be preferable. Socioeconomic and demographic characteristics of the population have been suggested as useful indicators, but the precise relationship between such variables and health status or needs is as yet poorly understood. However, standardized mortality rates (SMRS) are administratively feasible and, though a poor proxy for minor ailments, obstetrical needs, and mental illness, have been shown to be a valid indicator of the need for health care. In particular, they correlate well with those types of morbidity (for example, chronic or terminal conditions) that demonstrate considerable and continuing needs for health care.[44]

That SMRS can actually be applied to allocation of health care resources is clear from a 1993 study of the needs of Ontario's forty-nine counties. The researchers calculated equal per capita shares of Ministry of Health funds for 1989 and then adjusted them according first to the age and sex mix of the county population and then to the differential health risk of these populations, based largely on SMRS. The results suggested that some counties would receive dramatically more and some significantly less resources than would result from allocation solely on the basis of relative population.[45] The study obviously raised major issues, such as what geographical units should be used, what local authority should manage resources, how raw data on need are best collected, and, most important, how to deal with the opposition of regions that would see their resources diminished. SMRS are not the only useful approach to planning, as is illustrated by Quebec's more complex system, in which age accounts for 60 per cent of needs variation,[46] or by growing interest in use of geographical information systems to rationalize resource allocation.[47] Needs-based planning is clearly a trend that will grow in Ontario over the next decade.

Resources cannot, however, be distributed entirely according to seemingly objective measurements of need, and the allocation process must also take into account preferences that may on occasion correlate poorly with needs. The expression of preferences points to a fifth trend evident in Ontario health care – enthusiasm for community-based planning and resource deployment. Most recent Ontario reviews of the health system evince support for this notion, but it has received its most explicit endorsement from the Premier's Council on Health Strategy. This group strongly recommended that the government work towards 'devolving responsibility for the provision of health and social services ... Devolved responsibilities include: budgetary allocation; service management; service planning; service co-ordination; service monitoring and evaluation.'[48] The council assumed that empowering local communities would enhance efficiency by creating more accurate awareness of needs and would avoid often-inappropriate decisions coming from centralized authority. As well, it believed that this approach would allow for a more robust voice for vulnerable social groups.

This conception of the community's role in the health system is far more aggressive than that traditionally undertaken by district health councils and may reflect a deeper shift in social values. Specifically, it has been argued that citizens are less comfortable with decision-making delegated to bureaucracy, feel that governments are less legitimate, and reveal changing values that would be conducive to increased involvement and activism. Yet it is not clear how the popular voice might best be heard. Traditionally governments engage people along a continuum, which includes dissemination of information, consultation, partnership, less often delegation of power, and, rarely, citizens' control. To reach the last-named level for health resources requires both a means for the public to express its views and a method for organizing that voice.

Public views on health care might theoretically be solicited through continual issue-oriented polling, but the cost and logistical awkwardness limit the applicability of this technique. More practicably, members of the public speak through representatives of various sorts, including elected political officials; ascriptive leaders, to whom groups delegate speaking authority; descriptive leaders, who are assumed to be representative of the characteristics of the group from which an opinion is sought; and substantive representatives, who are selected on the basis of their recognized expertise on particular issues.

Organizing these spokespeople into effective structures for planning and management purposes presents another series of choices. At the least formal level are spontaneous grass-roots groups, composed of representatives or organizations that discern a common purpose, often a single, immediate issue. Such groups may coalesce with other similar bodies to form a network and eventually evolve into a more structured, broadly based citizens' coalition. More selective but perhaps more manageable are leadership boards, which bring together leaders from relevant interest groups for a specific purpose. Citizen panels are similar but tend to be used largely in a consultative role by government. Finally, a specific interest group may act as a lead agency to spearhead and direct community involvement and decision-making.[49] Each of these formats has precedents in the health sector, and, while the degree to which all members of the community are willing to participate remains problematic,[50] Ontario's restructuring health care system seems very likely to evolve a wide range of opportunities for local communities to plan and manage health resources.

The five trends in Ontario health care discussed in this chapter are not the only emerging themes in the province's approach to health,[51] nor is the manner in which they will find practical expression at all certain. But it is clear that these themes have already appeared in a large number of recent Ontario policy initiatives,[52] including attempts at long-term reform, hospital restructuring and amalgamation, introduction of alternative providers such as midwives and nurse practitioners, and experimentation with health-information data systems. Against a background of severe financial constraint, over the last decade Ontario's health care system has been subject to profound rethinking and restructuring. Physicians tend to be traditionalists and frequently isolated from the political and economic forces acting on the environment in which they practise. This chapter has described some of these forces and the manner in which they translate into trends in the management of health care. It shows that the physician-specific issues discussed in the following chapters are not the product of a focused attack on the profession, but part of an inexorable system-wide evolution.

2 Paying the Piper: The Fee-for-Service System and Its Alternatives

Canada's health care system combines its own traditional entrepreneurial fee-for-service format with the type of state-funded, universal-access system more characteristic of European nations. While it is doubtful that any health planner would deliberately set out to create such a hybrid system it is none the less the way things have evolved in Canada: private entrepreneurialism in symbiosis with public altruism. It is a system that puzzles US observers, whose responses have recently ranged from enthusiastic[1] to dismissive[2] and displayed highly divergent levels of knowledge and mythology,[3] often reflecting little more than the employment affiliation of the commentators. At home the system struggles in a period of ill-defined transition in which the issue of how to pay physicians looms large.

The present chapter presents an analysis of these seemingly strange bedfellows – entrepreneurialism and state funding. It begins with a description of contemporary attitudes and issues dividing government and the medical profession. Next, it seeks the origins of these disputes in the often-troubled evolution of medicare. It then compares the strengths of the fee for service system, both under Canadian medicare and more generally, and its acknowledged weaknesses. It concludes with a consideration of three alternatives for how Ontario's system might evolve over the next decade.

In Ontario, approximately one-third of the provincial budget is spent on health care. In 1980 the Ministry of Health budget stood at $4.9 billion; by 1990 it had more than tripled, to $15.3 billion.[4] As a proportion of provincial gross domestic product (GDP), health spending escalated from 4.7 per cent in 1975–76 to 5.5 per cent in 1989–90. A portion of this increase was a result of diminished federal transfer payments, which fell during this period from 1.6 per cent of the national GDP to 1.2 per cent.[5] Faced with a record deficit in 1992, the province was unwilling to spend more on health, and so from 1993 through 1996 gross payments to physicians actually declined slightly.[6] Years earlier, during the 1970s, medicare appeared to have curbed the rapid increase of physicians' fees that had characterized the decade before its inception.[7] But while the province remained modestly successful in curbing hospital costs[8] in the 1980s quite a different trend was evident for physicians' services. From 1983 to 1989 fee-for-service payments grew at 12.5 per cent yearly. In contrast, the number of service claims grew at less than half that rate, the number of new physicians at one-third that rate, and the number of services per physician at a scant 0.3 per cent per year.[9] Negotiated fee increases comprised a small proportion of the yearly growth, amounting, for example, to 4.83 per cent for 1987 and 1.75 per cent in 1988.[10] The government concluded that individual doctors were billing more aggressively for an approximately stable volume of service, leading to an unacceptable rise in payments to physicians.

In support of this interpretation, the Ministry of Health could point to a significant alteration in the billing practices of family physicians. For no obvious medical reason, between 1983–4 and 1988–9, use of the billing code for an intermediate assessment – approximately 50 per cent more lucrative than a minor assessment – rose by 13 per cent, with a reciprocal fall in minor assessments. Other billing indicators, such as the use of the code for emergency-department equivalent or for delegated services, such as audiometric testing, revealed a similar increase.[11] The effective result for general practitioners, excluding those billing less than $30,000 per year, was a 26 per cent increase in average payments from the Ontario Health Insurance Plan (OHIP) from 1984 to 1989.[12] Small wonder then that the ministry bluntly concluded: "Medicare's future is at a crossroads ... Ontario cannot support continued double-digit growth in health expenditures."[13]

On the other side of the fiscal debate are Ontario's physicians, who complain bitterly that "underfunding" of the system has deprived them of appropriate remuneration. In a 1987 national survey of physicians, three-quarters felt that doctors were losing economic ground, compared to other professionals.[14] These views receive some confirmation from statistics on relative income. While in 1959 Canadian physicians earned 3.7 times the national average of wages and salaries, two decades later this figure had fallen to 3.4.[15] This decline doctors attribute to the parsimony of medicare. Similarly, figures from the Organization for Economic Co-operation and Development confirm that physicians in the United States, Germany, and Japan during the mid-1980s had significantly higher incomes than Canadian doctors.[16] Canadian physicians are particularly envious of fees in the United States, which rose 22 per cent from 1971 to 1985, while those in Canada fell 18 per cent when adjusted for inflation.[17] The result has been that the net incomes of American physicians in 1987, though the product of a lower per-capita service rate, were one-third higher than those of Canadians.[18] This figure does not, however, take into account the far higher proportion of primary-care physicians in Canada, who, as in the United States, receive much less income than specialists.

By 1996 barely half of Canada's physicians indicated satisfaction with their incomes.[19] Particularly upsetting to the profession is the fact that, despite the high profile of the topic, payments to physicians have not grown more rapidly than payments in other sectors of health care. In Ontario the cost of laboratory services grew by 15.4 per cent per year from 1983 to 1989.[20] For all of Canada, from 1975 to 1985, the increase in the cost of physicians' services was exceeded by that of both dental care and drugs and comparable to increases for hospitals and other institutions.[21] Further, the cost of paying physicians accounts for a relatively small proportion – approximately 16 per cent – of the total bill for health care.[22] Given this situation, it is not surprising that Ontario doctors view themselves as the hapless scapegoats in a financially troubled system. Rather than arbitrarily curtailing payments to diligent physicians, they argue, the government should turn its cost-conscious attention elsewhere, to issues such as manpower planning, alternative funding formats, and utilization management. The medical viewpoint, particularly as it applies to the fee-for-service system, is usually at odds, philosophically and practically, with that of the Ministry of Health. How did this discordance evolve?

Had medicare appeared in Canada at the same time as Britain's National Health Service in the late 1940s, the subsequent relationship between physicians and government would have been vastly different. In the early 1940s, with medical incomes ravaged by the Depression, the Canadian Medical Association was in the forefront of the crusade for medicare.[23] Physicians in Canada traditionally collected approximately two-thirds of their billings, but during the 1930s they often chose barter, payment in kind, or waived fees completely.[24] With the return of prosperity in the 1950s, however, interest in state medicine was quickly forgotten. In Ontario, payments from increasingly popular doctor-sponsored carriers such as Physicians and Surgeons Incorporated and Associated Medical Services accounted for approximately half of physicians' incomes and doubtless significantly increased the proportion of bills collected.[25] During the dozen years preceding introduction of medicare in Ontario, published physician fees in Canada exceeded the consumer price index by 1.1 per cent annually, and collected fees may have been much higher.[26] Thus there was little economic incentive for physicians to welcome state-funded medicine.

The transition from a private to a publicly funded system in Canada has been described as "a series of short term bargains between power groups, similar to the British process of 'muddling through.'"[27] In 1969, with still-fresh memories of the acrimonious and protracted doctor's strike that greeted Saskatchewan's launching of medicare in 1962, Ontario bureaucrats appear to have adopted a deliberate policy of gradual, incremental change. Existing private insurance companies were allowed to act as carriers for the provincial plan. Physicians were reimbursed 90 per cent of the amount billed for each service, based on the existing tariff of the Ontario Medical Association (OMA), with the balance being held back to cover administrative costs. Physicians were allowed several billing options: they could charge all services to OHIP; they could bill the patient directly for any amount, and the patient later received reimbursement from OHIP at the 90 per cent rate; or they could charge OHIP 90 per cent and the patient the remaining 10 per cent or more.[28] As well, physicians were permitted to combine these options within their practices according to the perceived economic status of individual patients – a format referred to by physicians as "the Robin Hood principle." There was thus little that was frightening or unfamiliar for physicians in the early, flexible model of medicare in Ontario. Indeed, the guaranteed collection of 90 per cent of billing must have been extremely attractive. But the very ease with which the system began suggested that the real problems were yet to come.

From the physician's point of view, despite gloomy predictions, the early years of medicare were very lucrative. In 1970 medical incomes in Canada had risen to 4.85 times the national average income.[29] Almost immediately the Ontario government, with the establishment of its system no longer a subject of debate, insisted on changes designed to tighten administration and control costs. Its so-called practice-streaming rule, adopted in 1971, required physicians either to opt into the program, thereby accepting the 90 per cent OHIP payment as payment in full for all patients, or opt out, retaining the right to bill all patients directly at any rate, with the patient later receiving reimbursement at the 90 per cent rate. By 1972, 86.5 per cent of Ontario's physicians had opted in,[30] and the profession had effectively abandoned the right to price discrimination.

With the vast majority of Ontario physicians no longer able to vary their individual prices, the key element became OHIP's fee schedule. In recognition that it would be paying for piece work at a rate that it did not control, the government had in 1969 required that the OMA notify the ministry six months in advance of any proposed increase in the tariff. Joint discussion, informal by later standards, would ensue concerning aggregate increases, though deciding on the distribution of the increase within the tariff remained a prerogative of the OMA. The first increase occurred in 1971, but in 1973–74 a more formal mechanism, the Joint Committee on Physicians' Compensation, was created. This process proved unsatisfactory to the OMA, and in 1975 it refused to negotiate its tariff. Instead, it agreed only to negotiate a "schedule of benefits" for OHIP payments, which by 1980 lagged behind the OMA's tariff by about 30 per cent. At the same time, the OMA urged physicians to opt out so as to be able to use legally the OMA's tariff rates and greatly increase political pressure on the government.[31]

No mass opting out took place, and the OMA was brought face to face with what was rapidly becoming a monopsony. For its part, though it had exerted some cost control through fee negotiations, the Ontario government still found itself committed to paying for whatever medical services the public demanded from an increasing number of physicians willing to supply those services. The concerns of both government and physicians were crystallized by Parliament's passage of the Canada Health Act in 1984. Already with the passage of the Established Programs Financing Act in 1977, Ottawa had tied levels of its previously unconditional cost-sharing for medicare to growth in the gross national product. Now, with the 1984 legislation, it elected to withhold proportionate funds from any province permitting extra billing.[32]

Despite physician's virulent protests and withdrawal of services, Ontario passed its Bill 94 in 1985; doctors could still bill their patients directly, but not for an amount in excess of the OHIP schedule. Ontario had considered, like Saskatchewan, following Quebec's example of permitting physicians to practise entirely outside medicare without reimbursement for their patients. But the spectacle of Regina's ophthalmologists opting out en masse persuaded the Ontario government that the more stringent model used in Nova Scotia would be the only effective way to prevent emergence of opted-out pockets of impaired access to services.[33] The 1985 act effectively removed the one financial incentive for remaining opted out, since direct billing carried with it increased physicians' administration costs and the risk of nonpayment. As physicians had always feared, true monopsony had arrived; government was now poised to use its power to control costs more aggressively.

The medical profession learned important lessons from the extra-billing débâcle. The right to extra-bill, by topping up the incomes of economically motivated physicians, had reduced pressure on the government to increase OHIP fees. But equally, it had served to defuse discontent among OMA members over the relative distribution of fees within the schedule. Increasingly, office-based physicians would criticize the undue fee weight given to procedurally oriented practitioners. While some unregenerate doctors in Ontario tried to replace extra-billing with so-called administrative charges – that is, direct payment by patients for services not covered by OHIP such as phone advice, prescription renewal, and transfer of medical records – their enthusiasm was circumscribed by the judicious guidelines of the licensing authority, the College of Physicians and Surgeons of Ontario.

By 1987 the dust appeared to have settled. A national survey of physicians revealed that barely half still favoured extra-billing, while 60 per cent disapproved of withdrawing services and stated that they were satisfied with practice under medicare.[34] These results were interpreted as confirming the conclusions of a pre-Canada Health Act survey which suggested that only a minority of doctors, many of them leaders in medical associations, ideologically opposed medicare.[35] And even these individuals, sobered by their humiliating defeat in 1985, appeared ready to retreat from open confrontation over fees to enthusiastic attempts to find other ways of helping the Ontario government control costs. Economies in other areas of the health sector, it was doubtless expected, would translate into more liberal fee increases for physicians.

In such a climate of begrudging compromise, the time was ripe for the Ontario government to take the next step in cost control – a curb on use. The Canada Health Act forbade implementation of any user-fee deterrents. Some federal restrictions on immigration of foreign medical graduates were already in place, and postgraduate training programs in Canada were being gradually reduced in size, both aimed at reducing the supply of doctors. But the real focus of the problem occurred in the offices of physicians already in practice. Ontario did not appear to contemplate restricting the number of physicians eligible to bill the provincial plan as was attempted in British Columbia, or to legislate locations for first-time practice, as Quebec proposed. Instead, it introduced two mechanisms. First, in 1991 it capped specialists' incomes at $400,000, beyond which OHIP payments fell by 33 per cent; at $450,000, they dropped by 67 per cent. Physicians in under-serviced areas or those with a unique skill could receive exemptions. Of the seven hundred specialists affected, approximately fifty obtained exemption.[36] Second, and ultimately a more significant measure, though opposed by the OMA since first discussed in 1987, it tied fee increases to utilization rates – an approach already deployed in several Canadian provinces.[37] The government agreed to pay the first 1.5 per cent of growth above population and demographic adjustments, with the remainder of the increase in billing shared equally with the profession. This schedule resulted in a 1.2 per cent payback by practitioners for the first quarter of 1991.[38]

The new method, as soon became clear, did not achieve its stated goal. Indeed, because government agreed to pay a portion of the amount by which the aggregate payment was exceeded, the arrangement was a "soft cap," which could at best slow growth of payments. As a result from 1993 a "hard cap" allowed for payments exceeding the allocated aggregate budget to be "clawed back" entirely from the profession on a per-physician percentage basis. Firm caps are far more effective than soft ones, though there are difficulties if the cap level is too high or enforcement is lax.[39] Such regulations, as is the case with soft caps, create chronic strife within the profession characteristic of common-property resources, that is, individual practitioners seek to maximize their individual share under the existing budget, to the collective detriment of the profession.[40] Finally, caps create chronic conflict with government over the appropriate dollar level of both individual and collective caps, which readily spills over into other areas of policy as well. This point was dramatically emphasized in late 1996 when Ontario physicians overwhelmingly rejected a draft agreement negotiated between the Ministry of Health and the OMA because of limitations on physician's mobility resulting from restrictions on the distribution of the billing numbers that physicians need when they bill the province. A subsequent agreement ratified by the profession in early 1997 deleted such restrictions but maintained both thresholds on individual specialty-specific payments and a hard cap on aggregate payments.

In summary, the first quarter-century of medicare in Ontario seems to have brought the fee-for-service system to an impasse. On the government side, there is firm belief that the rate of OHIP payout must become first predictable and then subject to control. This the ministry has attempted to do by capping the incomes of individual physicians and linking the aggregate income of all physicians to levels of use. From the viewpoint of much of organized medicine, physicians' entrepreneurial autonomy has been unjustly abolished, medical incomes have failed to keep pace with other professions, and increased public demand for medical services is unjustly charged against physicians' incomes through the 'utilization formula.' From either perspective it would appear that the fee-for-service system faces major problems. Is it worth keeping?

The fee-for-service format does have certain strengths, the first of which is that it is congruent with the traditions and self-image of the medical profession.[41] It implies autonomy in matters of judgment or ethics, freedom to set conditions and volume of work, and emphasis on the principle that the physician serves the interests of the patient rather than of a third party. Such individual professional freedom moreover is seen as characteristic of the way in which all citizens of a liberal democracy, regardless of occupation, should be treated. Surveys of Canadian physicians establish that half believe that medicare has already impinged on professional autonomy and that such convictions are largely subjective, rather than a function of demographic characteristics of the physicians.[42] An American study has documented marked preference for a fee-for-service style of practice among primary-care physicians, when compared with a capitation format, for reasons that included greater professional autonomy, enhanced intellectual stimulation, and more appropriate use of time.[43] In Quebec, where government regulation has been more intrusive than in other Canadian provinces, two-thirds of physicians surveyed in 1981 found fee for service the form of remuneration most conducive to professional autonomy, and a majority considered it the best guarantee of patients' access to care.[44] If physician identity and status contentment are deemed at all relevant to the smooth operation of the health care system, the fee-for-service system appears the most appropriate payment method.

Second, the fee-for-service system, by providing economic incentives, clearly increases the volume of medical activity. This finding leaves aside crucial concerns as to whether such activity is necessary or desirable, which are considered below. Both a salary system and capitation do not offer physicians incentives to provide anything beyond a minimal level of service to patients.[45] In an American paediatric setting, for example, fee-for-service physicians, when compared to salaried doctors, were found to see their patients significantly more often.[46] Similarly, a fee-for-service system would seem to explain, along with other important factors, higher surgical rates in the United States and Canada than in England and Wales.[47] It is doubtful then that even those opposed to entrepreneurial medicine would quarrel with its claim to inspire a greater volume of physician services.

Third, no system clearly superior to fee for service has yet evolved. Relevant studies have compared American capitation-based health maintenance organizations (HMOs) to fee-for-service practice. There is no direct Canadian equivalent to HMOs, the closest approximation being Ontario's Health Service Organizations (HSOs), which emerged after 1973. The Ontario government curbed funding to these groups in 1991, and their numbers fell from eighty-eight to seventy-six over the next four years. A consensus seems to exist that HMOs are less costly, largely because of the dramatically lower rates of hospitalization for their patients,[48] though HSOs do not appear to share this characteristic. The quality of ambulatory care seems generally equivalent in both models.[49] Patient satisfaction, perhaps because of diminished contact with one physician, may be somewhat lower in very large HMOs.[50] Though it is often asserted that preventive care is more common with capitated or salaried practice, the existing literature remains divided.[51] As well, alternative funding, while it exempts the government from negotiating a fee schedule, brings with it the need to determine a wealth of new policies concerning capitation rates, risk penalties, ambulatory care incentives and so on, which requirement has been a chronic problem in Ontario.[52] No clear advantage then emerges for existing alternatives to fee for service.

Fourth, the fee-for-service system may be more congruent than alternatives with patients expectations. Identification with a single primary-care physician may decrease service use in comparison with the multiple providers often found in a capitated setting.[58] Continuity of provider care has also been shown to enhance patient appointment keeping and compliance with medications – both markers of the quality of care.[54] Some American studies have failed to document significant differences in patient satisfaction when comparing pre-paid and fee-for-service patients.[55] Yet the notion of a private contractual relationship between patient and physician, despite funding from a third party, implies a degree of intimacy traditionally perceived as central to the doctor–patient relationship. Lastly, on a pragmatic level, patients are sufficiently astute to realize that removing the economic incentives of a fee-based system may result in a slower response by physicians to a narrowed range of concerns.

It is difficult to identify other advantages for the fee-for-service system. In fact, the above points constitute a very tenuous argument in favour of retaining it. One could easily argue that a minor advantage in terms of providers' and consumers' preferences, a tendency to define output largely in terms of volume, and lack of persuasive data on alternative systems are hardly the firm criteria on which 16 per cent of a nation's health-care resources should be dispensed. This fragile position becomes even less secure when one considers current arguments against the fee-for-service system.

Critics of the system assert: "Fee-for-service payment ... is incompatible with the control of long-term global expenditures."[56] There are two major reasons for this incompatibility. First, in the United States, studies of fee freezes or reductions such as occurred under Medicare in Colorado between 1976 and 1978,[57] under Medicare in California from 1968 to 1976, and in a number of other locations[58] support the notion that attempts to control unit prices result in both increased use and greater complexity of services billed. In effect, physicians have implicit income targets that are relatively inelastic in relation to actual payment rates.[59] Suspicions of similar trends are found in Canada. Though physician fees from 1971 to 1983 lagged behind the consumer price index by 1.7 per cent yearly, use per physician increased at an annual rate of 1.4 per cent, a growth rate sufficient to offset all but 3.4 per cent of the income lag over a twelve-year period.[60]

Lurking behind such observations is the concern that rising use is a product of physician-induced demand – consumption of services that patients would not seek if they were as medically well-informed as their physician. Studies rejecting the view that fee for service leads to overconsumption are in a minority. In the United States data from the National Medical Care Expenditure Study estimated that 39 per cent of visits were physician-initiated,[61] while an Ontario study placed the rate at 20 per cent.[62] As the American study pointed out, many of these visits had clear origins in the health needs of the patients served, substantially reducing the proportion of visits attributable to physician income-targeting. Yet the data on rising medical charges in U.S. areas with increased density of fee-for-service physicians provides, contrary to expected supply and demand relationships, persuasive evidence of the ability of physicians to stimulate demand for their services independent of medical need.[63]

Second, personnel constitute an inhibiting factor in long-term control. While Canada has, when compared to the United States, been relatively successful, through use of negotiated fee schedules, in controlling increases in per-physician expenditure, a growth in the number of physicians billing medicare undermines this control.[64] In Ontario from 1975 to 1987 expenditures for physician services per physician increased 38.7 per cent reflecting a 17.7 per cent real price increase and a 17.8 per cent increase in per-physician use. Yet the number of physicians also increased by 26.1 per cent. The result was an overall increase in expenditures on physician services of 96.8 per cent.[65] Only in Quebec, which applied a stringent set of individual and collective payment caps, has evidence emerged for costs' increasing at a rate less than the growth in the supply of physicians.[66] Faced with such considerations, the influential report *Towards Integrated Medical Resource Policies for Canada* (1991) lamented that the expansion of physician supply in excess of population growth continues without obvious justification.[67] Many of its recommendations, such as an immediate 10 per cent reduction in medical-school enrolment and curtailing of the entry of foreign graduates to Canada, received rapid endorsement by provincial ministries of health. This issue will be considered at greater length in the next chapter.

Third, while cost control is a major problem for medicare with a fee-for-service format, so too is monitoring of the claims process for both overt fraud and over-servicing. It is a problem common to many jurisdictions, and the surveillance systems in place might be labelled, as in British Columbia, "cumbersome, secretive, and ineffective."[68] At best, monitoring may act as a deterrent, but most systems have an unimpressive record of convictions. Ontario established the Medical Review Committee in 1972. Though a creature of the provincial College of Physicians and Surgeons, it derives legislative authority from Ontaraio's Health Insurance Act, and both its lay and medical members are appointed by the minister of health. Initially OHIP attempted to screen practitioners using a quality-service payment formula based on estimates of the maximum billing that could be submitted by a physician without compromising quality of service. This system had a false positive rate in excess of 80 per cent and was abandoned in 1975.[69] Of the 519 cases referred to the Medical Review Committee from 1972 to

1976, 65 per cent resulted in recommendations for repayment of OHIP fees by physicians. At present, OHIP identifies aberrant or inaccurate billing patterns by computer screening, random audit letters to patients, and direct complaints from the public. If there are grounds for believing that billed services were not rendered, were medically unnecessary, were improperly rendered, or were misrepresented, the case is referred to the Medical Review Committee by the general manager of OHIP. Between 1988 and 1991, the committee completed 246 investigations, with 64 percent resulting in orders for recovery of funds totalling a mere $6.16 million. Despite reforms to expedite investigations introduced in 1995,[70] it is difficult to envisage an effective method of monitoring and detecting abuses under the current fee-for-service billing system.

Fourth, if the fee-for-service format does not lend itself to either cost control or surveillance for abuse, neither does it readily promote quality of care. In fact, the converse may be true. There is no incentive for physicians to discourage overuse or trivialization of medical services by patients. Thus, more than 12 per cent of funds spent in Ontario in 1991 on primary care were for minor upper respiratory infections, for which treatment is at best symptomatic.[71] Busy practitioners seeking to maximize volume may, when confronted with complex cases, order excessive investigations or inappropriately refer patients to a specialist. It is problematic whether this is preferable to a capitation system with a provider-risk clause, which may discourage investigation and referral, thereby endangering quality of care. Some physicians may be tempted to incorporate lucrative gimmicks, such as performing screening audiograms on all patients in their practice. As well, the fee-for-service system discourages physicians from delegating care to less expensive providers such as optometrists and chiropractors, even when this care might prove superior. Entrepreneurial considerations may clearly impinge on the quality of care.

Fifth, the issue of quality affects not only the patient's welfare but also that of the physician. The fee-for-service system fails to reward doctors for excellence of care, instead recognizing only volume of output. OHIP regulations make no provision for compensation for time-consuming tasks such as composing complete referral letters, renewing patients' prescriptions, dispensing telephone advice, and preparing detailed summaries for transfers of medical records. The contributions of those physicians who provide extended office hours, needed house calls, or excellent on-call service are not recompensed. Instead, less committed doctors may sign over evening responsibility for their patients to expensive walk-in clinics or refer patients to emergency rooms rather than make a home visit, thereby dramatically increasing costs to the system. Finally, the schedule of benefits under medicare in Ontario – the product of internal deliberations within the OMA – rewards procedurally oriented physicians, to the detriment of office practitioners. These anomalies, resulting, it has been claimed, in income differentials of 1500 per cent, have been labelled 'grossly unfair' and the adoption of a relative-value format has been urged to rectify the situation.[72] The OMA has attempted to devise resource-based scales of relative value,[73] but to date no changes have been introduced.[74] Thus quality care by a low-volume, office-based practitioner receives no monetary recognition under the current system.

Incorporating a quality-assessment element into any remuneration system poses significant conceptual and practical problems, considered in greater detail in chapter 5. In Ontario, quality of care is largely unmonitored and completely unrelated to payment. The province's College of Physicians and Surgeons operates a mandatory peer-review program, which randomly selects physicians for scrutiny of their practices, including patient records, to ensure that their standard of care conforms to the accepted norm. The College of Family Physicians operates a mandatory recertification program for those holding its credentials, but such qualifications are optional for general practitioners in the province. Some research suggests that certified doctors compared to other general practitioners, provide better care[75] and bill OHIP less per patient per month.[76] Within hospitals, attempts at quality assurance included departmental chart audits, tissue-review committees for surgery and monitoring of prescription patterns by pharmacy committees. No medical body in the province can enforce any obligatory continuing medical education, and cynics argue that only the tax-deductible status of such courses explains their use by the profession. In short, no effective mechanism currently exists for evaluating the quality of care dispensed by Ontario's physicians, regardless of their form of remuneration.

It is clear that the Ontario fee-for-service system has, through its troubled quarter-century of evolution under medicare, both failed to establish a persuasive list of advantages and is vulnerable to a wide range of criticisms. What then are future policy options for a system of physician remuneration? Three dramatically different alternatives are possible.

The first option involves essentially a return to earlier practices. As the federal government pursues its avowed policy of withdrawing transfer payments for health care, it will lose the only means of forcing provinces to abide by the Canada Health Act. Ontario will then be free to remove the prohibition on extra-billing so that physicians may "top up" OHIP earnings, and the province will also take the opportunity to impose user fees as a deterrent to excessive use of family physicians and emergency departments. Already certain items such as employment physicals or back-to-work certificates have been "delisted" by OHIP and physicians are free to charge patients any amount. As well, the province has introduced income-linked user fees for the Ontario Drug Benefit Plan. Such an approach would preserve physicians financial autonomy, ameliorate the Ministry of Health's funding difficulties, and diminish use of the system.

Unfortunately user fees have been shown to harm those least able to pay – the poor and the elderly.[72] In the case of drug expenditures, for example, co-payment provisions lead to reduced consumption of both non-essential and essential medications.[78] This option would also probably result in the gradual emergence of that most dreaded creature in the Canadian health planner's lexicon – a two-tiered system. As in Britain, physicians would be able to opt out entirely, and their patients would finance their visits completely through privately purchased insurance.[79] The resulting public system would co-exist with a small private version of the American entrepreneurial system. On equity grounds alone, it is doubtful that this alternative would have much appeal for Canadians.

A second vision of medicare's future is diametrically opposed to increased privatization. Rather, the provincial government, unwilling to depart from the bedrock principle of universal accessibility but faced with rising expenditures, will terminate the fee-for-service system. The process may be phased and negotiated or abrupt and arbitrary. Two possible methods have been discussed. The first is devolution of the Ministry of Health's planning and funding powers to regional authorities.[80] These bodies would have the power to determine the number, type, and location of physicians required and the rate and format of remuneration for those services. Doctors in excess of the numbers thought to be needed in the region would not have access to regional funding or institutional resources. A second but similar proposal is the comprehensive health organization (CHO).[81] It is a community-sponsored conduit through which ministry funds would flow for purchase of services that the organization identified as necessary for the care of its rostered population. A CHO therefore has the ability, like regional authorities, to determine the number and type of physicians that it requires and the payment format. In all probability general practitioners would be paid by a capitation method, while specialists would be hired on either a sessional or an individual-case basis.

While there are marked differences in the political implications of regional authorities and of CHOs, both produce very similar systems of physician remuneration. First, access to services is universal, unlike in a two-tiered system. Second, in theory these models accommodate legitimately identified needs thus reducing expenditures for surplus use. Third, these methods ensure control of physician numbers – a significant cost factor in the current system. Fourth, the funding authority can demand built-in quality-assurance mechanisms for all practices. Fifth and finally, the funding authority has the power to negotiate and budget for rates and methods of remuneration for the physicians it chooses to hire. In effect then these two methods of delivering services have the potential to control the cost, the volume, and the quality of physicians' services. They therefore appear the best long-term policy option, and many of their salient characteristics may eventually be merged under the more recent label "integrated delivery systems."

The third policy option, if the past is any guide, is the most probable, though by no means the most desirable – ad hoc, incremental "muddling through." Consider the following examples of incrementalism. The detente of 1996 between government and organized medicine stabilized Ontario's fee-for-service system and gave the government time to plan a more comprehensive approach to physicians' remuneration. Already the province is cooperating with physicians to delineate evidence-based guidelines for cost-effective care as the work of the Institute for Clinical Evaluative Sciences suggests.[82] Physicians and bureaucrats are pledged to scour the OHIP listings of services for those that are not medically necessary and can be shifted to privately financed care. Canadian attempts to define those "core services"[83] to be publicly financed are reminiscent of the now-famous Oregon experiment in rationing care.[84] Recognizing that physician numbers have traditionally helped determine aggregate cost, the government has reduced medical-school and postgraduate positions and restricted entry to practice to individuals trained in Ontario. All the above initiatives might be expected to help government deal with the issue of physician payment. But the critical solution will be more direct and will probably echo a decision taken in Britain at the inception of the National Health Service – paying specialists and general practitioners by quite different methods.

Specialists will probably be paid in one of two ways. Those consultants practising in the five Ontario academic health sciences centres will receive sessional payments through the type of alternative funding plans pioneered by the Department of Paediatrics at the University of Toronto and subsequently expanded by the Faculty of Medicine at Queen's University. The centres will receive envelope funding in return for providing secondary and tertiary care for a specific catchment area. Specialists outside academic centres may continue to bill on a fee-for-service basis but will be subject to specialty-specific thresholds. To make the process more equitable, both the Ministry of Health and the OMA are committed to creating a fee schedule based on the resource-based relative value of the services provided. Two other factors may prove important. First, province-wide retraction of the hospital sector will limit practice opportunities for new specialists in many locations. Second, the declared intention of delisting non-essential items from OHIP coverage may enhance the ability of specialists to augment their incomes by providing services not subject to threshold regulations. In short, outside academic centres the future would appear to promise fewer specialists providing fewer services, and subject to closely regulated income levels.

The situation for family physicians will probably prove quite different and, in many ways, more innovative. A variety of proposals have surfaced in recent years, all designed to separate primary care from fee-for-service billing. Some observers have advocated emulating the recent British system of "fund holding," under which groups of family physicians receive envelope funding from which to purchase all the medical needs of their rostered patients. Ontario's College of Family Physicians has since 1992 called for a "blended funding mechanism" comprised of a base salary, overhead costs, and both volume and non-volume modifiers.[85] Still others have suggested "publicly financed competition," under which government would finance both traditional fee-for-service physicians and capitation practices. Patients choosing the more costly option would be required to pay the difference.[86] None of these suggestions, however, is as compelling or as comprehensive as the OMA's proposal of 1995 for reform of primary-care payment.[87]

The key to the appeal of the 1995 OMA proposal is twofold: first, it incorporates interlocking incentives and disincentives for each group of stakeholders–physicians, patients, and government–designed in aggregate to encourage cost-effective use of the system; second, it retains many traditional, and therefore unthreatening, elements, blended with significant innovation. Each family doctor would have a roster of patients for whom he or she would bill on a fee-for-service basis up to a ceiling, defined by the number of patients multiplied by an annual capitation rate adjusted for the age, sex, and diseases of the patient population. This compromise system would discourage the under-servicing characteristic of pure capitation, while imposing a cap on each practice according to the size and needs of its patients. Government would find this method appealing as an alternative to a purely volume-driven system, particularly because annual budgeting for primary care would be possible once capitation rates were set. Patients would be required to sign on with a designated practice for a defined period such as three months, during which time they would pay directly for any primary care sought outside the practice. Physicians who failed to provide adequate service such as extended hours, phone advice, or on-call facilities would rapidly lose patients to those practices willing to meet patients' expectations. This feature thus curbs misuse of the system while requiring that physicians respond to the legitimate demands of patients who are at liberty to "vote with their feet" several times a year. This complex set of checks and balances on the behaviour of each stakeholder appears likely to emerge as the infrastructure for reform of primary care in Ontario.

What then can one conclude as to the fee-for-service system in Ontario? Such a method has been the dominant form of medical remuneration in most Western nations for the last two hundred and fifty years and has proven itself immensely adaptable to changing social circumstances. In Ontario, despite the introduction of medicare, it has evolved and, its critics would argue, thrived. To change it in any fundamental way would require an act of political will possibly beyond the capacity of a provincial government. Moreover, any change would demand as a prerequisite a clear demonstration that an alternative would provide equal care at lower cost. To date this possibility has not been established, with the preferred policy options as yet in the discussion stages. By tradition and default, Ontario's fee-for-service system lumbers on, transmuting and evolving, but with its essence always recognizable for what it is – private entrepreneurialism in awkward symbiosis with public altruism.

3 How Many Pipers?
The Supply and Distribution
of Physicians

James Henry, an Ontario physician active in medical politics, expressed the following views in a letter to a medical journal: "It must be apparent to every medical man in the province that the profession is becoming fearfully filled; that the number ... entering upon the study of medicine is greatly in excess of the wants or requirements of this young country."[1] The year was 1888, and Henry was expressing the traditional opinion of established practitioners competing with new graduates in recessionary times. Almost a century later a health economist considered the same issue in the following terms: "Because of the pivotal role of the physician in determining the utilization of medical, hospital, and almost all other types of health services, there is fundamental link between manpower planning and utilization or cost control. If, at the regional or national level, the physician stock is not a controllable variable, then all health budgeting is necessarily open-ended."[2] Here was quite a different emphasis on physician surplus: it was no longer simply a problem between practitioners; with the introduction of medicare, it had become an important issue of social policy.

Despite its clear importance over time, however, planning for numbers of physicians has not been an area of policy success. This chapter first assesses the current situation – it looks at growing fears that Ontario has developed a surplus of physicians, inadequacies in recent planning for medical personnel, maldistribution of physicians, policy levers open to government in dealing with a physician excess, and constraints limiting these options. It then examines possible solutions – restructuring of Ontario's health care system via devolution or comprehensive health organizations (CHOs) and a model for immediate intervention.

Does Ontario have too many physicians? There is as yet no precise method by which to identify an optimum number of physicians for a given population. Implicit in the following material, however, is an acceptance of the argument that a dramatic increase in the numbers of doctors relative to population increase in the absence of compelling proof of a commensurate and causal improvement in the population's health constitutes strong circumstantial evidence for a physician surplus.

There are, of course, counterarguments to this position. It can be shown, for example, that the ratio of physicians to population has increased less rapidly in recent decades than is the case for other health care workers such as nurses, pharmacists, and laboratory technologists.[3] It has been contended that Canada far from possessing a surfeit of medical students, may face a shortage of new doctors early in the next century.[4] Finally, it has been argued that increased numbers of physicians per capita have been necessary to meet the increased patient demand, which followed the introduction of state-funded health care.[5] Despite these contrary positions, and acknowledging caveats concerning specialty mix and geographical distribution, this chapter assumes that the weight of evidence favours those who perceive a surplus of physicians.

Since the 1950s physician supply has dramatically outstripped population growth in Canada, as it has in most developed nations.[6] While growth appeared to level off in 1990–1, for the period 1975–87 the number of physicians grew by 43 per cent, compared to population growth of 12.6 per cent.[7] This rapid growth was rooted in part in needs projections from the federal Royal Commission on Health Services of 1964. Seeking to preserve the 1961 population–physician ratio, but overestimating population growth to 1991 by almost 30 per cent, it recommended dramatically increasing the domestic production of physicians.[8] The implementation of its recommendations may have reflected the government's conviction that medicare would abruptly increase demand for physicians. But as early as 1971 two Ontario physicians were able to declare that the province's output of medical graduates, without augmentation from the foreign graduates then comprising about 60 per cent of new Ontario physicians yearly, would meet all needs for the next two decades.[9]

That a surplus loomed may have been evident to some prescient observers, but in the 1970s policy in Ontario failed to confront the issue directly. Instead, numbers of hospital beds were reduced as an indirect inhibition of medical practice, and the federal government in 1975 introduced some controls on the admission of foreign medical graduates to Canada. Yet the number of postgraduate trainees and newly licensed physicians continued to grow throughout the 1970s. It was not until 1980, after a second review of Canada's health care system, that Mr Justice Emmett Hall warned publicly of an existing physician surplus[10] – a sentiment overtly endorsed by Ottawa four years later.[11] As in the United States,[12] in Canada organized medicine was reluctant to concede a surplus and did not do so until 1989.

The medical personnel issue in Ontario came to a head in 1993. The immediate stimulus appeared to be publication of the Barer-Stoddart Report, an exhaustive study prepared in 1991 for the Federal, Provincial and Territorial Conference of Deputy Ministers of Health. It recommended a 10 per cent reduction in enrolment of undergraduate medical students, a policy that the Ontario government implemented almost immediately. It also suggested controls on licensing of graduates of foreign medical schools, a 10 per cent reduction in postgraduate training posts, and incentives to encourage new graduates to locate in under-serviced areas.[13] The Canadian Medical Association (CMA) countered with tepid proposals for cautious and gradual alterations to output from domestic medical schools.[14]

Few observers anticipated the precipitous announcement by the Ontario government in the spring of 1993 that new general practitioners, paediatricians, and psychiatrists would receive payment at 25 per cent of the established rate for five years if they insisted on establishing practices in the over-serviced areas of urban Ontario.[15] Nor were enough vacancies in under-serviced areas available to absorb all the new physicians entering the market. The government revised its intended draconian level of payment from 25 per cent to 75 per cent, but the proposal expired with the tenure of the

NDP government. Three years, later, however the Conservative government precipitated a similar storm of medical protest by announcing its intention to restrict billing numbers for new graduates to under-serviced areas. This policy was also abandoned, yet the acrimonious debates that followed these unilateral declarations of intention served no purpose more dramatically than illustrating the complete failure of effective medical personnel planning in Ontario.

Much of the planning failure in Canada can, as Jonathon Lomas and colleagues have argued,[16] be attributed to methodological and process limitations. Most planning has used as a starting point an inventory of current medical resources or levels of service provision, with the intention of projecting forward. There are major limitations to this approach. The data available on current medical personnel are often inadequate. For example, a 1980 Ontario study discovered that one-third of family physicians registered with the Ontario College of Physicians and Surgeons were dead, were retired or had left the province. Data in the past, even when translated into full-time equivalents, have failed properly to distinguish general practitioners from specialists or to consider those areas such as obstetrics or anaesthesia where there is significant practice overlap. Nor do raw numbers address the important issue of distribution of providers. As well, levels of service provision are assumed to reflect legitimate need, ignoring physician-induced demand or the significant proportion of services that are ineffective or inappropriate. The present, it is clear, provides a poor footing for the future.

Planning usually involves adjusting current figures, always upward, to accommodate any short-fall in providers. These alterations are done on the advice of experts, inevitably physicians and usually from academic centres. Not surprisingly, they tend to display particular concern for the future of their own or related specialties, and, despite the absence of any evidence of competence in the planning process, their opinions are generally accepted.[17] Moreover, these ex cathedra statements never include consideration of options such as the education of physician substitutes, which would decrease the need for doctors. Rather, factors such as an ageing population or the feminization of the medical labour force, which would tend to increase the need for physicians, receive central emphasis.[18]

The now-adjusted personnel figure derived from current conditions is finally projected forward to ascertain target physician to population ratios. The figure takes into account attrition rates for physicians and immigration from out of province, balanced against assumed rates of population growth. Other factors, such as an ageing population, introduction of new technologies, and changing behaviour of physicians such as women general practitioners (who work 87.7 per cent of the number of hours claimed by male physicians[19]) are taken into account. These calculations yield a target number to which medical education directs itself. It fails to consider a number of key variables, including consumers' changing preferences, the impact of prevention strategies, real or potential structural alterations such as changes to remuneration systems or the provision of physician substitutes, disease prevalence and impact, and standards of optimal treatment. Small wonder then that future medical workforce figures are little more than inaccurate projections of current resources, filtered through the selective prejudices of the projectors themselves. The end result appears to have been a dramatic increase in the physician surplus.

Perhaps in recognition of the problems associated with past efforts to plan for the future need for physicians, the mid-1990s witnessed a flurry of planning activity. The provincial and territorial health ministers, for example, announced in 1994 their joint intention to develop a schedule for the development of a national plan for physician supply.[20] In the same year provincial and territorial medical associations, together with the Canadian Medical Association (CMA), formed the National Ad Hoc Working Group on Physician Resource Planning. The report of the group[21] endorsed several departures from past planning exercises. For example, it suggested use of the notion of a "critical mass" of doctors, rather than simple population-to-physician ratios, so as to ensure adequate coverage in rural or remote areas. It also recognized the need to categorize services so that esoteric specialties would not be expected to be distributed on a geographically equitable basis. But despite acknowledgment of the importance of developing needs-based planning tools, its approach relied on population-to-physician ratios in a manner all too familiar to those aware of the earlier critique by Lomas and his colleagues. In summary, governments and medical groups have done little to address current and future concerns about a growing physician surplus.

Despite reasonable evidence for a doctor excess, it is widely argued that the current distribution of physicians is inappropriate in that it fails to provide necessary medical personnel for northern or rural areas. While figures for Ontario are often imprecise, it is known that the physician-to-population ratios found in northern counties such as Timiskaming (1:840), Kenora (1:839), or Rainy River (1:880) are twice those found in southern metropolitan areas. More sophisticated measures of distribution are location quotients, which use the ratio of a region's number of physicians to that of the entire province in comparison to the ratio of the region's population to the province's. A value of less than unity indicates under-representation of medical personnel. Using this method, a study of the fifty-two counties of Ontario revealed that in 1986 none of the ten northern counties exceeded a quotient equal to 0.8, while in the south nine counties had quotients below 0.5, and twelve had values below 0.749.[22]

Unequal distribution of physicians is by no means unique to Ontario. In 1992 in Canada as a whole, 23.5 per cent of the population lived in rural areas, yet only 17 per cent of family physicians and 4 per cent of specialists practised in these areas.[23] In 1985 in Manitoba, 78 per cent of the province's physicians practised in Winnipeg which had a physician-to-population ratio of just under 400, compared to 1,130 in the rest of the province.[24] In 1990 in Alberta large urban areas possessed 65 per cent of the province's inhabitants, but 78 per cent of its physicians.[25] As well, in the United States it has been estimated that one in seven Americans live in regions with a critical shortage of primary-care physicians.[26] Even in the highly planned British system, several recent studies document that general practice resources[27] are poorly correlated with areas of documented need.[28]

The precise significance of this unequal geographical distribution is much less clear than its existence. Is equity of access defined by distance to the nearest physician, per capita supply of physicians, per capita use of resources, or availability of "necessary services"? Access is obviously influenced by many factors in addition to numbers of physicians, including availability of alternative providers, practice patterns of physicians, the formal organization of the medical system, and the age and gender of the population. To date there is no sustained outcry from rural or northern areas regarding general access to physicians, nor do morbidity or mortality rates document dramatically unmet needs. Indeed, needs-based evidence is almost entirely lacking,[29] which factor, when coupled with poor data on current medical personnel levels, results in highly subjective target ratios for physicians to population.

To achieve equity in Ontario between isolated northern regions and the more populous south, the province has deployed two policies – the first implicit, the second explicit. The first, implicit policy has been dubbed the "trickle down approach" and rests on the assumption that if the overall supply of physicians in the province increases dramatically, a significant number of the new recruits will naturally gravitate to under-serviced areas, where they face less competition. There is no evidence to suggest that this process has occurred in Canada,[30] though Ontario's physician population increased from 8,040 in 1961 to 19,481 in 1985.[31]

The second, explicit policy in Ontario has been almost entirely under the auspices of the Ministry of Health's Under-serviced Area Program. Established in 1969, by 1987 it sponsored 575 physicians in two hundred communities and boasted an annual attrition rate of less than 5 per cent. Potential recruits are solicited during medical school, where a year of service is demanded for each year of subsidized education. Failure to comply results in the student's refund of medical-school expenses plus interest to the ministry. New practitioners receive $40,000 free of income tax, paid quarterly, over four years. Many communities are assisted to build clinic space and housing, which are made available to new physicians at very low rents. The program operates a *locum tenens* program to provide some leave time for its recruits, sponsors travelling specialists on a per diem basis, and in some locations operates nursing stations, which are visited periodically by physicians.[32] Despite these laudable efforts, rigorous assessment of the distribution of Ontario's physicians in 1986 concluded that, despite some changes, northern Ontario was as relatively underserviced as it had been in 1956.[33]

What policy levers are currently available to government to deal with the maldistribution and surplus of Ontario physicians? The first step is to stem the flow of new physicians, by restricting admission to licensure of graduates of foreign medical schools by negotiated alterations in both federal immigration policy and licensing provisions of the College of Physicians and Surgeons of Ontario. As well, reductions in both undergraduate and postgraduate training positions, a process already well under way, could be systematically pursued.

As education cutbacks take place, a second but related policy option might be initiated – the training of physician substitutes. Already the Ontario government has established a midwifery program. Additionally, it has been estimated that a significant proportion of visits by primary-care physician could be delegated to nurse practitioners with no loss of quality or patient acceptance. Over a twenty year period, it has been suggested such practitioners in Ontario could replace up to one-third of general practitioners.[34]

In addition to the above policies relating to education, a second policy lever exists – alterations to the method of paying physicians. Already in place in Ontario are caps on the aggregate billing of the profession, together with separate caps for individual specialties and family practice. These provisions may act as a deterrent to financially motivated physicians to locate in Ontario. The province has considered restricting the quantity of billing numbers in the province, in a manner calculated not to succumb to a court challenge, as happened in British Columbia. During its five years in existence, there was evidence that the BC law curtailed growth of that province's physician supply.[35] Finally, Ontario has recently declared its intention to introduce a system of differential fee payments for new physicians, which may be sufficiently stringent as to preclude recent graduates from establishing practices in the urban south. Simulation techniques have clearly demonstrated that income manipulation can alter both specialty mix and community of location.[36]

A third policy lever concerns efforts to redistribute Ontario's physicians. First, attractions must be offered to persuade new graduates to practise in remote areas. The Ministry of Health could ensure that medical schools recruit qualified students from underserviced areas who are most likely to return to practice in such locations. As well, medical schools must ensure undergraduates and postgraduates exposure to practice in rural areas.[37] Attention must be given to ameliorating conditions of practice, which the CMA has suggested are the primary concern of doctors in remote areas. Isolated practitioners could be assisted to locate in group practices with defined on-call obligations, regular study leave, and specialist back-up.[38] Secondly, restrictions in the form of limitation on access to hospital facilities might preclude specialists from locating in over-serviced areas.[39] Finally, alternatives to the actual relocation of physicians might be considered, such as improved patient transportation services, ranging from emergency air-lifts to routine clinic visits via scheduled buses.[40] Together, such policies would correct or compensate for the maldistribution of physicians.

The above policy levers are available without any fundamental restructuring of Ontario's health care system, but what countervailing constraints currently face government planners? The first problem confronting policy analysts is a paucity of relevant data. Refinement of sources such as the CMA's Physician Resource Databank and the Ontario Physician Human Resources Data Centre at McMaster University has made available information on the number, location, and functional status of physicians.[41] But data on regional health status, essential to needs-based allocation of physicians, are sadly deficient.[42] Moreover, data linking interventions to health outcomes are generally scant, thereby inhibiting researchers' ability to assess whether the cost of additional physicians would be justified by improvements in the population's health.

A second major planning constraint is the politically sensitive link between supply and distribution of physicians. As discussed above, despite an active Under-serviced Areas Program in Ontario since 1969, current data suggest that the ten northern counties are markedly underserviced. As a result, any program that attempts to curtail aggregate physician supply in the province, without also correcting for maldistribution, will be perceived as impairing access for northern citizens.

A third major area of constraint is the organizational and structural inertia of the current system. There are at least three distinct factors involved. First, medical schools' output cannot be rapidly altered: a first-year class enters practice six or more years in the future. Second, the fee-for-service system in the province, as in most Western nations, has been the dominant mode of medical remuneration. As discussed above in chapter 3, it is a central component in medicine's self-image as a profession of altruistic but independent entrepreneurs. Any plan to control physician supply by adopting capitation or salaries across the board would meet substantial medical resistance. Finally, though the profession recognizes a collective obligation to protect the public interest in a clinical sense, it often evinces little appreciation of its duty to a larger public or social interest.[43] The argument that the profession is a creature of the society in which it exists and must subordinate its concerns to those of a collectivity beset by financial constraints will thus not strike a resonant chord. In concert, the weight of established practices in medical education, professional remuneration, and practitioners' ideology constitute a major obstacle to changes.

A fourth and final constraint is difficult to document but concerns implicit public attitudes. According to surveys, Canadians highly value their health care system and are resistant to significant change that they fear would impair access. This attitude in itself inhibits change, but beneath it lies a larger faith in medical science. It is a naive notion, which also assumes as axiomatic that more, like new, is better. Thus, for example, persuading a public nurtured on the liberal mythology of scientific progress that fewer rather than more magnetic resonance imaging (MRI) facilities might improve population health is difficult if not impossible. Scaling down the system will inevitably be equated with diminished quality through diminished access and more limited resources.

Could restructuring help solve the physician surplus? It is clear that the legacy of inadequate planning methods has led to a critical and costly physician surplus in Ontario. As well, the distribution of physicians is far from optimal. While policy options are available under the current system, some may be slow to show effect or certain to provoke vitriolic conflict with organized medicine. Moreover, their ability to effect change is counterbalanced by a series of structural and ideological constraints of considerable magnitude. It therefore is necessary to consider whether extrication from this policy dilemma lies beyond conventional approaches, in new and innovative restructuring of health care. In particular, do proposals for either devolution or comprehensive health organizations (CHOs) appear to offer practical improvements in the planning and deployment of medical personnel?

Proponents of alternative formats of health care delivery argue that such structural changes will, through the application of needs-based planning, allow accurate estimation of the number, specialty mix, and distribution of physicians to meet identified health goals within a defined population. Needs may be identified through a variety of indicators, including case registries for specific disorders, population surveys, standardized mortality rates, demographic variables such as age or gender, and indicators of social deprivation such as unemployment.[44] While such data could be collected at the provincial level, some observers argue that local information-gathering increases accuracy and relevance. Moreover, advocates of alternative means of delivery emphasize community decision-making in the needs-identification process.

This points to an important but neglected semantic issue. The term "needs" carries with it an implication of value-neutrality, of validity independent from the observer. In fact, beyond nutrition and shelter, designation of a resource as something needed is simply a subjective process of attaching particular urgency to a preference. Further, not all identified needs can be gratified, which necessitates a setting of priorities – another clearly subjective process. It is recognition of this subjective component within needs identification that provides the rationale for local community planning, which is thought to be preferable to centralized decision-making. Most planners, however, agree that the provincial government should retain a role in specifying certain minimum province-wide requirements and standards for provision of services.

Current models of devolution in health care propose a local authority to identify needs and deploy resources to meet them. They accomplish this goal through transfer from the Ministry of Health of not simply a funding "envelope" but also the authority to allocate it in any reasonable fashion.[45] The proposal for southwestern Ontario, for example, envisaged a regional health board responsible to the ministry and selected in an unspecified manner. It would have six area health-management boards reporting to it, as well as a use review board. The proposal stated: "Physician resources which are beyond the needs of the Region will not be given access to the health system in Southwestern Ontario."[46] It envisaged incentives to encourage redistribution of doctors, alternative funding formats, increased use of physician substitutes, and negotiations with the local medical schools to ensure adequate preparations of graduates for practice in non-urban areas.

Specific plans for implementation of devolution were conspicuously lacking. It is difficult to imagine any scheme that would uproot existing practitioners, and so the current surplus of urban physicians is likely to remain for some time. The distributional aspect of physician supply would be immediately amenable to alteration by precluding practice by new graduates in undesignated locations. Since the regional authority was to decide the dollar amount to be spent on doctors' services, it could easily manipulate remuneration rates to encourage changes in the aggregate supply of practitioners as well as specialty mix. It is clear then that devolution could exert a powerful positive effect on planning for the physician workforce. But if this goal is considered in isolation, is such a radical transformation in Ontario's delivery of health care actually necessary?

A less dramatic policy suggestion is the development of comprehensive health organizations (CHOs), a term adopted by the Ministry of Health in 1988.[47] A CHO is a community-based organization that acts as a transfer agency for funds from the ministry. It provides a specified range of services to a defined population using existing health delivery resources, which either merge with or contract to the CHO. The CHO is obliged to provide all required services, as dictated by the identified needs of its population and as mandated by the ministry. But the allocation of dollars to meet these needs is at the discretion of the CHO itself. Primary-care physicians will probably be paid on a capitation basis, while the services of specialists in all but very large CHOs would likely be purchased on a contractual basis. Because both spending authority and identification of needs rest with the CHO, levels of personnel can be readily controlled and altered for the CHO's designated population. In some areas of the province, CHOs might not be feasible, leading to a residuum of fee-for-service practice. As well, in areas where CHOs operated, some practitioners might refuse to participate or be surplus to their needs. They could continue to practise on a fee-for-service basis. However, their access to facilities such as hospitals controlled by the CHO could be curtailed, and the CHO, by providing superior service, could ensure no loss of its subscribers to independent practitioners.

Both devolution and CHOs appear able to control physician personnel. They both allow community authority for planning, promise more accurate local data, encourage cost-effective integration of services, and permit manipulation of personnel resources to achieve desired goals. They also share weaknesses. Regions or CHOs may provide different levels and ranges of services, leading to spillage of consumers into other catchment areas.

Local planners may have less expertise in designing large-scale systems and be more susceptible to the influence of powerful local interests. In some regions there may be disproportionate influence accorded health-science centres. There may also be a discordant relationship with the provincial government over a wide range of issues.

The question remains, however, as to whether the widespread introduction of CHOs or regional authorities offers a method superior to the current system in controlling the physician workforce. The current system offers rapid, albeit insensitive methods such as restrictions on billing numbers for abruptly inhibiting the growth of surplus physicians in already over-serviced areas. The alternative systems are years away from operation, a time lag that may witness dramatic growth of the problem. The current system, by making practice economically viable only in designated areas, can also rapidly assist underserviced areas. The new models are capable as well of redistributing personnel, but at a slower pace. Under the present system, the provincial government can effectively control the size of the province's medical schools, initiate the training of physician substitutes, and negotiate with the federal government to curtail the entry of graduates of foreign medical schools. None of these functions could be effectively addressed by CHOs or regional authorities alone or in concert. Public support for the current system is chronically high. Alternative systems, though clearly improving consumer input, risk being perceived as both coercive in any rostering requirement and as a disguise for providing lower levels of service. Despite all the recent turbulence, physicians would probably prefer the current fee-for-service system, which, rightly or otherwise, they believe preserves a greater degree of professional autonomy.[48] Finally, the current system to date has failed to introduce any needs-based workforce planning. While CHOs and regional authorities would probably prove more adept at this task, there is no reason to believe that the Ministry of Health could not effectively pursue this goal. On balance, while CHOs and regional authorities have long-run advantages, the current system appears capable of achieving rapid control of physician personnel in the short to medium term.

What might a policy for immediate intervention include? Given the geography of the province and current or future population distribution, variations in physician distribution are inevitable. But some improvement is possible. The following proposal, based on a number of sources and similar in part to Quebec's, where its success seems clear,[49] assumes continuation of fee for service in the short and medium term, combined with increasing emphasis on needs-based regional planning:

1   immediate introduction of a differential fee scale for new physicians for the first five years of practice, which pays 70 per cent in high-density areas and 130 per cent in under-serviced areas;
2   additional incentives to practise in remote areas, including subsidized clinic facilities, continuing medical education, specialist back-up, *locum tenens*, and on-call limitations;
3   immediate and progressive reduction in the number of both undergraduate and postgraduate training positions, with consideration given to the feasibility of moving one medical school to northern Ontario;
4   mandatory exposure for undergraduates and postgraduates to under-serviced areas, with specified residency slots in high-demand specialties being reserved for those committed to practising in remote areas;
5   the initiation of an intermediate- to long-term planning process to define physician requirements for specific geographical regions within the province.

This project would incorporate multiple methods on behalf of many stakeholders, including needs-based assessments, consumers preferences, and physician-to-population ratios. The results would be used to designate areas as over- or underserviced, according to specialty and would be compatible with alternatives to traditional fee-for-service practice. The success of such policy would create an environment for medical personnel more amenable to the introduction of CHOs or regional authorities. To these more radical alterations could be left the long-term task of creating a system that reflects needs or preferences rather than mere serendipity.

In conclusion, the sorry state of physician personnel reached in Ontario in the 1990s is the legacy of methodological and process deficiencies dating to the inception of medicare. While there are notable constraints on the present system, including poor data, professional inertia, and public prejudices, there are effective policy levers immediately at hand. The provincial government can control the domestic output of physicians and, by using differential fees and other tactics, control the distribution of that output. While both regional devolution and CHOs offer a superior long-term capacity to control the number and deployment of physicians, neither alternative is clearly superior to the present system in the short run. Indeed, one is left with the impression that what has been lacking until now in the current system is simply the political will to redress the neglect of previous years. However distasteful this task may prove in practice, it appears that its time has come.

4 Calling the Tune: Quality Assessment and Assurance in Ambulatory Care

Each month the Ontario Health Insurance Plan (OHIP) processes in excess of ten million claims. A large proportion of these are submitted by physicians for "ambulatory care encounters" – patients' visits to a doctor. The individual claim identifies the patient, the physician, the principal diagnosis, and the fee code for the service. Barring an administrative anomaly such as an incorrect numbers for the patient health card, the claim is generally paid without further inquiry. From that moment on, the encounter ceases to interest the Ministry of Health other than in its role as one minute contribution to the ever-increasing expenditures on health care.

But has the taxpayer received quality medical service? The traditional assumption has been that the medical profession, through its stringent educational standards and the policing role inherent in self-regulation, ensured that qualified practitioners dispensed a service of consistently high quality. Yet a growing body of evidence suggests that this belief is naive. At one extreme, for example, are studies that document adverse outcomes from medical interventions and estimate the proportion of these results attributable to negligence.[1] Beyond documentation of such overt mistreatment, however, lies the more vexing question of variance. Consider several examples. For the period 1966–76 surgical rates in Canada, for instance, were 60 per cent higher than those in England and

Wales, and the United States had higher and rapidly increasing rates.[2] Even within Ontario, surgical rates varied substantially by county between 1973 and 1977.[3] Population characteristics, conditions treated, and availability of health-care resources do not adequately explain these observations. Similarly, studies of internists have demonstrated extreme variation in the use of laboratory tests in the case of similar patients. Yet the pattern of test ordering failed to correlate with either the physician's clinical competence[4] or patient outcomes.[5] Recently the hospitalization of patients with acute myocardial infarction in Ontario has been shown to result in significantly variable lengths of stay, which are largely unrelated to patients' or hospitals' characteristics.[6] If physicians in each of the above examples presumably are committed to delivering high-quality patient care, how does one account for the variations in diagnostic and therapeutic approach? Which pattern truly exemplifies quality care? The inescapable conclusion appears to be that the quality of medical care, despite the good intentions of practitioners, is highly variable.

This chapter examines the assessment and assurance of quality as they apply to ambulatory care in Ontario; it does not consider in-hospital practice, where quality-assurance programs are more common and certainly more enforceable. First, it reviews existing attempts to assess quality in ambulatory care. Second, it examines some of the many constraints on assessing quality in outpatient settings. Third, it briefly discusses the major methodological options for both quality assessment and assurance. Fourth, it offers general suggestions as to how at least some aspects of a province-wide system of quality assessment and assurance may evolve in the near future and outlines five policy areas that might be addressed. The contention throughout the chapter is that regardless of imperfect methods to assess it, our present system is inadequate and must be rapidly and substantially revised.

As the agency charged with paying the bill for ambulatory care, OHIP might be expected to make some attempt to determine the quality of the services that it purchases, but does it actually do so? As discussed in chapter 1, this was the case for the brief period from 1973 to 1975. Ontario's Ministry of Health, in close consultation with physicians from each specialty, developed "quality service payment formulas." The formula represented an attempt to estimate the maximum volume of service that a practitioner in a given specialty could deliver without compromising quality of care. This procedure failed to reduce the number of false positive referrals for investigation and was quickly abandoned for a less cumbersome format.[7] At present OHIP simply identifies aberrant billing patterns by computer screening, sending random audit letters to patients, and responding to direct complaints from the public, with a minuscule number of cases resulting in demands for restitution.[8] An attempt to gauge or ensure quality is no longer in evidence at the ministry.

What role have professional credential-granting and educational organizations played in assessing quality? In Ontario, general practitioners are not required to hold the credentials of the College of Family Physicians of Canada (CFPC). Many family doctors, however, are certificants of the college and as such are required both to accumulate a minimum number of approved study credits annually and to sit a recertification examination every five years. Ambulatory care is also provided by specialists, all of whom are fellows of the Royal College of Physicians and Surgeons of Canada (RCPSC). Only recently has a pilot program for maintenance of competence (MOCOMP) been established by the latter body, and it is as yet far from obligatory. Collectively these educational programs are entirely voluntary and are not designed to ensure that practitioners knowledge is actually translated into quality practice.

Voluntary professional organizations are beginning to show an appreciation for the issues of quality of care. The Canadian Medical Association (CMA) formed a Quality of Care Committee in 1990. It undertook a survey of needs and existing resources across Canada, surveyed the attitudes of practising physicians, and published a useful literature review.[9] The Ontario Medical Association (OMA) has enthusiastically endorsed the notion of quality assurance through the elaboration of clinical guidelines.[10] It sponsored the formulation of guidelines for the use of thrombolytic agents in acute myocardial infarction[11] and, in conjunction with the Ministry of Health, for the detection and management of asymptomatic hypercholesterolemia.[12] Publication of such material, though professional compliance remains unmonitored, undoubtedly enhances physicians' awareness of quality issues.

In 1981, the College of Physicians and Surgeons of Ontario (CPSO) initiated an ongoing peer review process, under which practitioners are selected randomly for compulsory review. The physician is visited by practitioners from the same specialty, the practice facilities are examined, a number of charts are selected at random for detailed review, and the physician is interviewed by the reviewers. From 1981 to 1985, 918 physicians were assessed, revealing that 15 per cent of general practitioners and 2 per cent of specialists had serious deficiencies in either or both record-keeping and patient management. Among general practitioners, deficiencies correlated with advanced age, solo as opposed to group practice, and non-membership in the CFPC.[13]

For those physicians with identified deficiencies, the CPSO entered a joint venture with the OMA and the five Ontario medical schools to create the remedial Physician Enhancement Program.[14] Beyond this practical approach to remedial intervention, the CPSO in 1993 joined other provinces' licensing authorities to create an ongoing project entitled Monitoring and Enhancement of Physician Performance.[15] Yet the method currently in place in Ontario for monitoring quality of care – often dubbed "the bad apple" approach – focuses solely on the outliers among practitioners, thereby leaving unaddressed measures to assess and improve the quality of care among the province's competent practitioners.

Quality is, of course, an elusive concept, which makes its assessment all the more difficult. Most authorities would agree that at least two general aspects of quality are important in medicine.[16] First, care must be both appropriate – that is, neither unnecessary nor neglectful – and readily accessible. Second, it must be effective, physically and/or psychologically, in terms of outcomes for the patient. But even if this general definition is agreed on, applying it to the assessment of ambulatory care is fraught with difficulties. Some, though by no means all, of these dimensions may be captured under four headings – practice settings, therapeutic outcomes, chronicity, and the "art" of care.

Hospital care may occur in settings ranging from a cottage hospital to a tertiary-care centre. But the ends of this spectrum differ more in scale than in character. In contrast, ambulatory care takes place in widely different settings – community health centres, employee health offices, walk-in clinics, hospitals' out-patient departments, solo or group practices, emergency departments – to name but a few common venues. The type of records kept will show little uniformity of format or content, in contrast to standard hospital charts, making audits of records difficult.[17] The demographics of the patient population served may, unlike the undifferentiated population that uses a community hospital, be restricted by age, gender, or type of illness, making generalizations problematic. Finally, the location of ambulatory care ranges in Ontario from itinerant northern clinics to large urban practices next door to hospitals. This diveristy in turn influences access to specialists and diagnostic facilities. Given such a range of settings, finding commonly applicable criteria for quality assessment will prove difficult and will be compounded by the complex issue of who should bare the cost of such assessments.

It is often said that in medicine less than 20 per cent of what physicians do in routine practice has been shown to be of clear value through well-designed clinical studies.[18] While this statement probably exaggerates the proportion of unvalidated activities done by doctors, it does suggest how difficult it is to assume that clinical outcomes, good or bad, are necessarily the result of medical care.[19] In a primary-care setting this problem is magnified by several other factors. First, most acute illnesses seen by general practitioners are self-limiting and will resolve themselves spontaneously regardless of treatment of whatever quality.[20] Second, patients exercise considerably more autonomy in ambulatory-care settings than in hospitals. They may choose not to comply with recommended therapy or refuse appropriate investigations or consultations, decisions which in turn influence outcomes. Finally, a significant proportion of ambulatory practice requires no therapeutic interventions at all, but rather is devoted to disease prevention, an activity whose outcome is extremely difficult to measure.

Many of the clinical encounters in ambulatory care involve chronic conditions. The slow evolution of these disorders makes measurement of outcomes difficult, while in many general practices the scant number of diagnoses for any one disease makes evaluation of the management of that disorder statistically impossible. Considerations such as this have led to a variety of suggested methods by which quality of care may be inferred. For example, rather than observers waiting for a practice, as its patients age, to accumulate strokes or myocardial infarctions and evaluate care of the cardiovascular system on this outcome basis, they may use management of a common, known antecedent condition such as hypertension as proxy. A number of other techniques of varying validity are available for attempting to gauge the influence of medical intervention on the quality of life for those with chronic disorders. For many of the chronic conditions seen in ambulatory practice, however, the impact of medical care may be too subtle to permit accurate assessment of its quality.

In recognition of such difficulties, some researchers have suggested that assessments of ambulatory care must evaluate the far more elusive entity popularly referred to as "the art of medicine." One study of primary care concluded: "The most striking result ... was the absence of any relationship between the resolution of the patient's symptoms and the adequacy of history taking, physical examination, use of diagnostic tests, prescription of drugs or maintenance of a problem list." What did have explanatory power was "agreement between patient and physician about the nature of the patient's problem" – in short, communication.[21] As another study, however, has shown, family physicians may have excellent communication skills yet be weak in their diagnostic or therapeutic knowledge, which may have an offsetting effect on patient out-comes.[22] How precisely these various attributes are related to the quality of patient care remains problematic, though a growing literature on patient satisfaction suggests that the "art" of medical care is highly valued by its recipients and may to some extent reflect quality.[23]

Thus, there are significant problems associated with quality assessment in ambulatory care. The process must begin, though, with the conviction that whatever schema is selected will be superior to none at all and will itself be subject to continuous quality surveillance and improvement. Traditionally, estimates of quality focus on the triad of process, outcomes, and structure.[24] First, process in ambulatory care would include physician's accessibility, waiting time for appointments, duration of visits, content of various types of visits such as annual physical exams, mechanisms for obtaining prescription renewals or telephone advice, booking of referral appointments, and availability of house calls. Process would also include evaluation of diagnostic testing in specific clinical situations, prescribing of medications, appropriateness of physical examinations, and the arrangements for follow-up of patients and their test results. Second, the structure of care includes the physical environment in which the physician practises, available office equipment from waiting rooms to laboratory, the presence of clinical and administrative support staff, the appropriateness of phone systems and answering services, and arrangements for physician on-call coverage. Third, outcomes include death, disease, disability, discomfort, and levels of patient satisfaction or dissatisfaction.

A variety of methods have been devised to assess each of the three categories (process, ouitcomes, structure) mentioned above – most notably, "implicit" and "explicit." Perhaps the oldest technique, essentially that used by the CPSO's Peer Review Program, is the implicit approach. Skilled physician reviewers observe the subject physician in action and/or review the management of clinical problems as depicted in office charts. This method tends to rely less on strictly formulated performance criteria and depends to a much greater degree on the reviewers' global assessment. Its critics argue that it introduces undue reviewer bias and that assessors from outside the specialty of the physician under review are not true peers. To reduce the effect of bias, such programs usually deploy several reviewers, which makes the method very costly. This tactic has revealed that, in addition to there being documented intra-reviewer discrepancies, inter-reviewer anomalies are common. Finally, the results of implicit reviews do not always correlate with those using more objective methods.[25]

The explicit method of evaluation encompasses a continually expanding number of techniques. It uses specified criteria by which, through records audit, direct observation, and patient questionnaires, it assesses quality.[26] Billing pattern audits have also been used.[27] The process is less costly than implicit review because nonprofessional staff may do the evaluation. It also permits representatives of the specialty to be reviewed to help create the criteria to be applied – a major constituent of physicians' subsequent acceptance.[28] Yet it is an approach not without problems. The written medical record is not always an accurate reflection of what transpired at a patient encounter.[29] The format laid down to ensure that the necessary data will be found on even the most hastily compiled chart can be simplistic to the point of useless for quality assessment. An innovative solution has been "criteria mapping"[30] – an attempt to replicate in the evaluative criteria the branching logic of real-world clinical decisions.[31] As well, the assessment can choose to focus on a very specific "sentinel" item such as the follow-up of a positive test result that does not require scrutiny of an entire clinical encounter.[32] Even physicians who strongly endorse evaluative criteria, often fail dramatically to adhere to them.[33] This fact suggests that the criteria are unable in some major way to capture the complexity of clinical decision making.[34] Decision analysis is a method that may assist those designing criteria reflective of actual practice as it applies to individual patients.[35] Finally, it is unclear whether criteria formulated by physicians necessarily reflect the values and expectations of patients. This deficiency may be compensated for by study of patients' satisfaction,[36] often in combination with other endpoints such as self-assessment of level of functioning in everyday life.[37]

Assessing the quality of medical care is a necessary preliminary to assuring and improving quality. There are at present two general approaches to the complex task of assurance: establishing widely accepted guidelines, adherence to which will allow all practitioners to dispense excellent care, and the audit of practices to identify deficiencies amenable to improvement through educational feedback. The former tactic is increasingly popular, though opinions on its merits are divided. In 1990, for example, the US Congress created the Agency for Health Care Policy and Research, an agency equivalent to the Centres for Disease Control and to the Food and Drug Administration, to develop clinical guidelines.[38] As of 1991, thirty-two US physician organizations had published eleven hundred guidelines, and an additional 150 were in progress.[39] What is the role of such instruments?

Practice guidelines are strategies for patient management for specified clinical conditions or situations designed to ensure optimum quality of care. While some authorities are cautiously hopeful about the utility of practice parameters, which they view as an inevitable response to rising health costs and rapidly evolving medical technology,[40] others point to the failure of current programs. The Consensus Development Program of the National Institutes of Health, which has served as a model for Canadian activities, appeared to have no impact on practice in a large study in Washington state for such serious conditions as breast cancer and coronary-artery bypass surgery.[41]

Though some studies have found the consensus process sensitive to evidence,[42] others argue that guidelines often reflect little more than the personal bias of those making the recommendations.

Thus they may reveal opinions derived from tertiary-care teaching centres rather than from the average practitioner's office. Nor are they immune to economic considerations: guidelines endorsing lucrative procedures are more likely to be accepted by practitioners than those condemning such activities.[43] Even academic judgment has been criticized for failing to keep pace with very recent developments reported in the literature, resulting in inadequate or outdated recommendations.[44] Many guidelines are simply published, with no attempt made afterward to gauge their impact or effectiveness.[45] Finally, receptivity to guidelines may vary with the age or geographical location of the physician audience[46] as well as the perceived intention of the documents.[47] At least until these problems are addressed, such entities seem inadequate to ensure quality in ambulatory medical care.

While practice parameters can provide guidance but not necessarily guarantee compliance, the more costly and time-consuming process of practice audit seems substantially more effective. Though the current literature is somewhat ambivalent,[48] efforts to alter inappropriate use of x-rays[49] or drug-prescribing habits appear generally resistant to passive measures such as supplying corrective medical literature. But personal visits from clinical pharmacologists[50] or fellow physicians,[51] as well as introduction of the sanction of non-payment for inappropriate prescribing,[52] have been shown to alter prescribing patterns. Attempts to diminish excessive use of laboratory or diagnostic procedures show a somewhat similar response. While some educational interventions can influence physicians behaviour,[53] simple audit of a physician's resource utilization accompanied by educational feedback has been shown to be less effective than active chart review by other physicians.[54]

Finally, audit can alter patterns of clinical activity. A Harvard group has shown in several studies[55] that even unusually well-qualified practitioners reveal a substantial quantity of deficient care. In a randomized, controlled trial audit provoked serious efforts, despite resulting increases in costs, to correct deficiencies in those areas that physicians felt were within their control.[56] Simple feedback, though enhanced by both the speed with which it is made available[57] and a format-measuring performance against peers,[58] does not seem effective. Ongoing consultation with evaluators[59] and conversion and recruitment of local medical "authority figures"[60] will significantly prolong and augment changes in clinical practice. Auditing techniques in which physician evaluators or educators play a prominent role appear moderately effective in improving the quality of drug prescribing, laboratory use, and patterns of clinical practice.

The preceding pages have established that there is a recognized and as yet unmet need for review of the quality of Ontario's ambulatory care; that monitoring quality in ambulatory settings raises unique methodological concerns; and that both implicit and explicit techniques exist for assessing process, outcomes and structure and that practice guidelines and practice audit may enhance quality assurance. The balance of the chapter outlines how one might expect policy makers to resolve Ontario's quality conundrum in the near future and then suggests five areas in which it should develop policy.

The essential first step in elaborating an effective policy of quality assessment and assurance is recognition of the Ontario government as the pivotal authority. The province has an obligation to its residents, who are both taxpayers, who may want to know that expenditures yield proven value, and patients, on behalf of whom the province purchases health care, the quality of which must be guaranteed. In the United States, governmental responsibility for quality assurance has been a legislated part of Medicare since 1982 through Peer Review Organizations, successors to the earlier Professional Standards Review Organizations and the Experimental Medical Care Review Organizations.[61] Despite such precedents, persuading Ontario physicians that the government has a place in the process may prove difficult. Organized medicine tends to justify its own initiatives over quality as blocking possible government intervention. As well, American studies have documented the lack of actual participation and cooperation of physicians in quality-assurance programs, whatever their professed attitudes.[62] Yet open recognition of the provincial government as the leader in quality assurance is critical.

To this end, the province of Ontario should enter into cooperative ventures with existing medical groups, including the OMA, the CPSO, the CFPC, the RCPSC, and the medical schools. This process is already under way. For example, the Joint Management Committee, composed of OMA members and Ministry of Health officials, has directed major aspects of the province's health system since 1991. It has created the Institute for Clinical Evaluative Sciences to assist in evaluating approaches to medical care and technology, the results of which will provide a basis for evidence-based practice guidelines[63] similar to those previously issued jointly by the OMA and the ministry.[64] In another joint project, OHIP, in its review process, has since 1972 been identifying those physicians who appear to be billing inappropriately. Its general manager then refers the case to the Medical Review Committee of the CPSO. Its members are appointed by the minister of health and include non-medical representatives. In effect, a government agency works with a medical organization to identify and punish illegitimate billing activities, at least some of which affect quality of care. In yet another example, funding for community health centres and health service organizations now includes quality-assurance provisions. If the recent report of the committee reviewing the Public Hospitals Act is an indicator, the provincial government intends to legislate in fine detail mandatory quality-assessment and, -assurance criteria for publicly funded health facilities.[65]

This starting point for an effective program of quality assessment and assurance in Ontario is the recognition by government and medicine of both the government's leadership and its partnership with the medical profession. Such activities aim to enhance the health status of the province's residents. Three specific goals must be attained if Ontario is to reach this objective. First, any program must be fair to providers. Without the participation of both medical organizations and individual practitioners, no scheme will prove viable. In fact, the degree of overt participation in activities such as guideline formulation and auditing of practices will be the principal criterion by which this goal may be assessed. Second, the program must ensure better care for patients. Often an "information deficit" renders them unable to judge accurately the quality of their care. As a result, quality assurance has traditionally been delegated to medical organizations, but a public agency with less mixed allegiances would be preferable. The success of such efforts could be evaluated by criteria such as the incidence of adverse drug reactions and the number of deficient practitioners identified by peer review. Finally, a high-quality system of health care must accomplish the same tasks as our present system at less cost. By definition, a system in which quality is assured refuses to fund inappropriate or ineffective interventions, a category that encompasses an unknown proportion of current medical practices. The criteria by which this goal could be evaluated would include expenditures by the Ontario Drug Benefit Plan, use of laboratory services, and aggregate OHIP expenditures.

Within this general framework, the Ministry of Health should address policy in five specific areas – service payment, medical education, practitioner audit, alternative practice formats, and patient education.

First, there is considerable truth to the observation: "The most efficient way to eliminate inappropriate care would be to stop paying for it."[66] A link between service payment and quality assessment is currently found in the United States for Medicare and Medicaid and was implicit in Ontario in the approach of many private insurers prior to 1969. It would require an alteration in the present OHIP billing format and possibly the use of obligatory random audits. Ideally it should have an educational component, in which the current annual profiles of practitioners, which show an individual's service statistics in comparison to peers, could be expanded to include laboratory use and prescribing patterns under the Ontario Drug Benefit Program.

Second, the Ministry of Health should ensure that the five provincial medical schools include specific courses on quality assurance in the curriculum at both undergraduate and postgraduate levels.[67] It should also work with the directors of continuing medical education for the CFPC and the RCPSC to sponsor conferences and workshops that would become compulsory for those seeking ongoing accreditation.

Third, the province should provide funds to the CPSO so that it can develop and expand its peer-review program to cover more physicians yearly and cooperate with the OMA in developing explicit criteria and methods for evaluation. This CPSO–Ministry of Health link is crucial: physicians will cooperate more if they feel that their organization is part of the evaluative process, and the CPSO's involvement permits licence revocation for those refusing participation or resisting remedial intervention. Moreover, guidelines sanctioned by the CPSO assume an authority that may permit malpractice litigation for failure to conform.

Fourth, new approaches to delivery of health care that depend on provincial funding, such as community health centres and health service organizations, must incorporate sophisticated quality-assurance programs. For example, there has recently been interest in comprehensive health organizations (CHOS). It has been argued that the emphasis on organizing and coordinating the care of each individual would not only make care more convenient for patients but would also lead to greater efficiency, enhanced efficacy, and lower cost.[68] The report of the Southwestern Ontario Comprehensive Health System Planning Commission[69] stresses management of the health-care system so as to attain goals identified by the community in the most cost-effective manner. District authorities would have power to determine their physician resource requirements and to insist on evidence of appropriate use and quality-assured practice.

Fifth, patients should learn to demand quality medical care. This objective involves complex issues of education of patients, and social marketing, as well as the study of patients' preferences and the components of patients satisfaction.[70] Of concern is evidence that patients and physicians may view an office visit with quite divergent levels of satisfaction, based on very different criteria.[71] But what better ongoing system of quality assurance could be devised than the need to satisfy the appropriate expectations of an informed clientele?

Over a quarter century ago, Mildred A. Morehead, an American pioneer in assessment of the quality of ambulatory care, wrote: "The two major questions that arise when studies of the quality of medical care are considered are 'What is quality medical care?' and 'How can it be adequately measured?'"[72] Clearly the answers are as germane, though as elusive, today as they were in 1967. Yet Ontario's health care system can not await a definitive answer. We must, to quote the prominent American authority Avedis Donabedian, "make every effort, through research and development, to create a new science of parsimonious care, one that is more efficient without being less effective."[73] Only by beginning now can we hope eventually to solve rather than deepen the quality conundrum for the province's ambulatory care.

5 Restructuring the Pipers' Workshop: Physicians in Hospitals

Within the hospital, a familiar institution in the Canadian social landscape, no figure is more clearly visible than the physician. Indeed, the hospital has often been referred to as "the doctors' workshop." Yet this is a misleading metaphor. Unlike the artisan in his or her workshop, the hospital doctor pays no rent, hires no staff, buys no raw materials, owns no tools or equipment, and is guaranteed full payment by the state for whatever services are rendered, regardless of outcome. The failure of the workshop metaphor, in fact, points to the central anomaly of the physicians' role in the hospital – while doctors generate an estimated 60 to 80 per cent of hospital expenditures,[1] they are independent entrepreneurs rather than hospital employees and are often unaccountable to the institution for their costs and many of their activities. This chapter examines the consequences of this paradox and suggests ways in which it might be changed.

The chapter begins with consideration of two broad concerns that challenge the physician's role in hospitals. The first issue – escalating costs and a funding formula that does not encourage efficient care – is fuelled in part by treatment decisions made by hospital physicians. The second issue – highly variable utilization rates – also directly reflects patterns of medical practice. The remainder of the chapter argues that hospitals must define their role more clearly so that they can restructure the physician–hospital relationship in a manner likely to lower costs and improve utilization. It postulates first that hospitals must negotiate their service role with their clientele, rather than allowing it to evolve in an *ad hoc* fashion as a by-product of the interests of medical staff. It suggests as well that integrating physicians into the management structure of hospitals can reduce costs and improve care.

The growing cost of hospital care is a phenomenon for which physicians must take significant responsibility, since their actions and decisions are said by Canadian administrators to produce two-thirds of all institutional expenses.[2] Doctors and their patients in Canada, more so than their American counterparts, clearly have a taste for institutional care. Between 1976 and 1988 the number of hospitals nationwide increased by twenty-seven to 1,052, the average length of stay increased by over 12 per cent, and occupancy rose from 78.5 to 81.4 per cent of capacity. To finance these increasingly popular institutions required an average annual increase in per capita spending from 1975 to 1989 of 8.9 per cent, though the amount spent remained a constant 3.4 per cent of Canadian gross domestic product (GDP). In Ontario, hospital expenditures as a proportion of GDP actually dropped slightly, but the $7.4 billion spent in 1992–3 represented over 43 per cent of the Ministry of Health's total expenditures.[3] A variety of factors such as an ageing population, the availability of expensive new technologies, pay equity legislation, and large wage settlements, are predicted to increase future hospital costs.

In contrast to the American model, Canadian hospitals are financed almost entirely by public funds. Until 1969 in Ontario line-by-line budget negotiations between the Ministry of Health and individual institutions decided the amounts. After this date, a prospective global budget assumed a uniform percentage-increase formula. By pegging the rate below the level of inflation, the ministry could control the growth of hospitals and inhibit proliferation of programs. Administrators typically first made internal spending cuts and only then attempted to secure additional funding or postpone retrenchment.[4] Since the system was based on budgets extant in 1969, it may simply have perpetuated existing inequalities. Despite its inclusion of a growth formula, it did not adequately take into account growth in populations served or changes in the type of patients admitted. Finally and most important, the global budget system offered no significant incentives for cost-effective care and did not necessitate collection of the patient-level data likely to facilitate such efficiency.[5] In recognition of these inadequacies, Ontario in 1988 launched the Transitional Funding Initiative, which let a portion of a hospital's grant reflect the type and severity of cases treated.[6]

Despite its inequities, the funding format did achieve a crude control of hospital expenditures. In the period 1967–81, total expenditures in Ontario increased by only 16 per cent in terms of real inputs, as compared to 101 per cent in the United States. Real inputs per admission actually decreased by 1.21 per cent yearly in Ontario but grew by 4.15 per cent in American institutions.[7] This general trend continued throughout the 1980s, when inputs per admission in Ontario grew at 2.4 per cent and per patient-day at 0.46 per cent yearly. Most of the cost increases beyond general inflation were the result of hospital wages, which rose at a rate exceeding the general economy.[8] The global budget format imposed a form of implicit rationing; it did not encourage hospitals to provide more efficient or appropriate care. While the province could boast of providing care comparable[9] to American hospitals at a much lower cost,[10] there was clearly a need for change.

The Ontario government recognized that simple expenditure control had to give way to a more managed system. In reviewing hospital spending in 1991, it isolated a series of issues demanding detailed attention. It would review programs and services to eliminate duplication and create a more equitable distribution of workload. It would eliminate underused capacity that remained fully staffed and operational, and it would vigorously discourage retention of long-term care patients in acute-care beds. Hospital funding mechanisms were to be again revised, and hospital operations rationalized in terms of productivity, inventory management, and shared services. In this broader process, the province chose three key areas of physicians' cost-generating behaviour for close scrutiny and modification – admissions and length of stay, utilization rates, and patient servicing.[11]

Use of hospital resources in effect became the key to cost control. As referred to briefly in chapter 4 above, heightened awareness of major variations in use of health care resources to achieve seemingly comparable ends focused research attention on this issue.[12] Though clear evidence for differential use of laboratory resources exists,[13] surgical cases in particular lend themselves to more precise scrutiny. In thirty-two districts of Quebec, ten common surgical procedures studied over a three-year period were found to demonstrate three- to five-fold variations in use, which figures were unrelated to proximity to teaching hospitals.[14] Similar results were noted for Ontario's forty-four counties for eight procedures over a five-year period and could not be explained by variations in the supply of beds or surgeons.[15] For American Medicare patients, surgical rates for 123 types of operation have been noted to vary at least three-fold for more than half the procedures.[16] Canadian surgical rates have been shown for the years 1966–76 to be 60 per cent higher than those for England and Wales and American rates markedly exceeded both the United Kingdom and Canada.[17] In the United States no correlation was apparent between the use rate of several diagnostic or surgical procedures and the rate of clearly inappropriate use.[18]

Observers have suggested many factors as contributing to the observed variations in the use of health resources of which three are now considered. First, there are system-wide influences, such as the presence or not of a state-sponsored system of universal health care, the availability/accessibility of health care facilities such as hospitals, and the number, distribution, and types of physicians.[19] Second, there are physician factors, which may include type of training,[20] prevailing local practice traditions,[21] types of practice organization,[22] geographical location,[23] and sensitivity to a variety of non-medical pressures on practice styles.[24] Third, there are patient factors which include direct demand,[25] age,[26] medical need,[27] gender,[28] and socioeconomic class.[29]

Even if the causes of specific types of variation are identified, a second level of quandries remains: in a situation of differential use, how does one determine which rate is too high and which too low? In other words, can outcomes be linked to patterns of variation? Unfortunately, measuring outcome as a function of resource consumption is a relatively unrefined field,[30] focused on linking death, disease, disability, discomfort, and dissatisfaction to both the structure and the process of care.[31] Major investigations such as the Medical Outcomes Study in the United States appear promising.[32]

As well, the American government has established the Agency for Health Care Policy and Research, which initiated research into six conditions – angina pectoris, benign prostatic enlargement, gallstones, arthritis of the hip, uterine conditions and low back pain – which together give rise to more than half of all in-patient surgery.[33] Such efforts over time should assist in forging an objective linkage between specific approaches to clinical problems and expected results. This knowledge in turn may significantly reduce variations in use of health care resources for similar patients with similar conditions.

Pleasing though such prospects are, hospitals face the immediate task of reviewing and validating their current resource consumption. To achieve this goal administrators turn to the relatively new field of "utilization management," a process that compares institutional performance to appropriate clinical service standards and develops methods to correct deficiencies. It makes the assumption that clinically meaningful groups of case mixes should provoke predictable clinical responses, with a consistent pattern of resource consumption. A 1989 survey of 123 Canadian hospitals revealed that 80 per cent had some form of utilization management program, usually created in response to high occupancy rates or funding difficulties. While two-thirds of administrators felt that physicians supported their efforts, most were unsure what impact the programs had on both quality of care and rate of unnecessary admissions.[34]

These administrators were quite correct in their assessment of Canadian utilization management – in contrast to the American situation, few empirical data exist to support its effectiveness. Because global budget financing has controlled costs in Canada more effectively, there has been less pressure to study utilization. As well, initiating such programs entails very significant and often difficult changes in the relationship between administrators and medical staff.[35]

Yet there are exceptions, an early example being the Greater Victoria Hospital Society, in Victoria, British Columbia, which initiated its program in 1985. By 1987 it had created data that permitted peer review to identify differences among doctors for patterns of resource use in comparison to caseload and severity. It also used clinical leaders to develop practice guidelines acceptable to colleagues to serve as performance benchmarks in concurrent reviews.[36] The resulting program – Vi-Care – appeared to contribute to a reduction in admissions and patient-days and decrease admissions of the less severely ill. While concurrent influences were also present, it also helped reduce the number of chronic patients in acute-care beds and enhance the development of outpatient surgery.[37] Though as yet underdeveloped in Canada, utilization management seems to offer a potent tool for hospitals seeking to justify the consumption of increasingly scarce resources.

Canadian hospitals, it is clear, face financial constraints and must monitor the appropriateness of resource use. Each institution must clearly define its role in the community. This delineation process represents the first of two major changes in the part that physicians play in hospitals. Traditionally what a hospital did was largely a serendipitous reflection of the talents and interests of its medical staff.[38] This staff in turn was assembled by chance, largely as a product of random applications from new physicians for admitting and other privileges. In most Canadian hospitals such applications are reviewed by a credentials committee – a group of doctors reporting to a medical advisory committee (MAC). The credentials committee checks the accuracy of an applicant's claim to specific credentials and determines whether these qualifications are commensurate with the type of privileges requested. Except in the case of fraudulent or clearly inappropriate requests, credentials committees have usually recommended that the MAC grant the privileges, and it then would so recommend to the hospital board, where contrary views are seldom expressed.[39] Little attention was usually paid to the impact of appointments on the role and resources of the institution. The traditional model views application to the medical staff as an exercise in credentials verification rather than personnel planning.

Two basic changes are necessary, both of which will alter the traditional medical role. First, the hospital's functions must become more than a fortuitous by-product of medical staff interests, dignified by the lofty generalities of a board-generated "mission statement." Instead, a rational and uniform process must be applied to the addition of medical people to the hospital roster. The urgency of this need was recognized in Ontario in 1988 after a study of twenty-three hospitals showing chronic deficits. An absence of personnel planning was a common characteristic among these delinquent institutions leading the report to call for obligatory medical personnel planning and "physician impact analysis." Partially in response to this recommendation, the Ontario Medical Association, the Ontario Hospital Association, and the Hospital Medical Records Institute (later called the Canadian Institute for Health Information, or CIHI), established a task force to develop guidelines to assist hospitals in these activities.

The resulting publication[40] recommended two methods of assessing the effect of a doctor's appointment to a hospital staff. The first, the survey method, asks each hospital department to estimate the impact of the proposed physician's caseload on its workload and resources. It depends on an accurate projection of the new caseload, requires time and resources to complete, and creates incentives for department heads to overestimate cost, yet it may yield the most precise and detailed estimate of likely costs. The second method allows the hospital to apply the CIHI data on types of cases and intensity of resource utilization per case so as to estimate the relative cost of caring for the new physician's projected caseload. It allows comparison with other institutions that have added such physicians but does not indicate the impact on outpatient services. It is not known how many Ontario hospitals routinely analyse physician's impact. Moreover, studies to date comparing cost predictions generated by these two methods against subsequent actual costs found little correlation, largely because of inability to anticipate cost, size, and type of physicians' caseloads.[41]

Physician impact analysis may yet provide a valuable estimate of how a new practitioner will affect a hospital's resources. As such it would serve as an objective way for administrators to assign priorities in resource deployment, which will shape the hospital's role in the community. But impact analysis, while potentially superior to unplanned proliferation of medical staff, can never do more than indirectly affect a hospital's role delineation. A more effective method is suggested in the 1992 report of the committee reviewing the Ontario Public Hospitals Act. It recommends that hospitals, under the mediating auspices of district health councils, negotiate their role with community stakeholders in the form of a "social contract." This agreement would set out the services that the hospital would provide, demonstrate how these coordinate with those provided by other sources, and be congruent with the hospital's long-term plan. Signatories would be the hospital board and, on behalf of the community, the Ministry of Health, with neither side able to modify the agreement unilaterally and a formal dispute-resolution mechanism incorporated into any proposed legislation.[42] Under this system fortuitous additions to medical staff would all but disappear, to be replaced by deliberate decisions on physician resources designed to honour the institution's social-contract obligations.

Two other trends – devolution and comprehensive health organizations (CHOs) – may supersede revision of the Public Hospitals Act to ensure that hospitals effectively fulfil their roles. First, the concept of regional devolution is well illustrated in the 1991 report of the Southwestern Ontario Comprehensive Health System Planning Commission. This group proposed that the Ministry of Health provide a funding "envelope" but delegate to a regional health management board all other functions, including long-term planning, allocation of operating funds, approval of capital expenditures, and management of human resources. Under this model, hospitals' roles would be clearly defined, staff needs scrutinized, and services coordinated among institutions.[43] Second, the concept of CHOs envisages "envelope funding" for a given roster of patients. The CHO defines precisely the health needs of the group and either hires practitioners who work in facilities leased or owned by the CHO or purchases their services on a contractual basis.[44] Again, centralized planning to meet the health needs of a designated constituency is the essential feature. Both approaches would dramatically alter the tendency of hospitals' services to reflect primarily the interests of their staff physicians.

Defining the role of a hospital is an essential first step in addressing current hospital difficulties, but a second major change must follow – restructuring physicians' contributions to the daily operation of the institution. In this context physicians have traditionally behaved in a highly autonomous fashion, reflected in and encouraged by traditional hospital organization. Individual clinical departments are represented on the MAC which, through a chief of staff, reports directly to the hospital board. The MAC spawns a variety of physician-staffed committees to deal with admissions and discharges, infection control, pharmacy and therapeutics, medical records, and so on. The chief executive officer of the hospital also reports directly to the board and sits atop a parallel organization of administrative departments, support services, and professional services, such as nursing and physiotherapy.[45] These two organizational streams are largely separate rather than symbiotic in their functions. Despite increasing attempts to encourage cooperative effort by ensuring a role for doctors in goal-setting, cost containment, program development, and utilization review,[46] physician and administrators too often fall into separate camps, with highly divergent priorities.

This lack of communication reflects the pervasive though intangible clash within the institution between medical and management cultures.[47] While physicians depend on individual professional autonomy, managers pursue integration of diverse individuals into a cohesive organization. Doctors define themselves and their hierarchy through overt standardized credentials, but hospital bureaucrats are of diverse and often unknown backgrounds. For these managers, the hospital is the exclusive focus for their occupational skills, while for most physicians it is an addendum to office-based practice. Doctors submit, albeit often reluctantly, to collegial control, but managers are schooled to support an organizational hierarchy. Physicians have little tolerance for constraints on practice activities, whereas bureaucrats consider rules, procedures, and priorities essential to the harmonious functioning of an institution. As well, hospital managers are able to adopt a macro perspective, which encompasses the hospital and the community that it serves, while physicians have a micro perspective, focused entirely on individual patients. Finally, doctors can point to a very tangible outcome – the recovery or demise of a specific patient – whereas the output of most managers is less well-defined and often subsumed in larger processes. These two divergent professional cultures create a chasm between frequently uncommunicative camps. Mediation strategies that take into account these characteristics[48] and identify common goals and obstacles[49] are an essential prerequisite to a unified assault on hospital problems.

In the United States the differences between managers and medicine have been viewed by some scholars as symptoms of a deeper structural division between "professional monopoly" and "corporate rationalizers." The former group – largely physicians and biomedical researchers – pursues autonomy and control over the conditions of work, seeing delivery of health care as secondary to the proliferation of clinical departments or research programs. The rationalizers, represented by hospital administrators, public health authorities, and government agencies, preach cost control, coordination, and integration as the basis for inexpensive, accessible care. They favour placing doctors on salary, restricting access to expensive technology, and enhancing the authority of their own bureaucracies.[50] During the 1970s the rationalizers were joined by private American corporations, whose rapid invasion of the hospital sector caused it to grow faster than the computer industry.[51] The new corporate power over hospital physicians has been referred to as the "proletarianization" of the profession,[52] and it might be argued that an analogous government-induced process exists in Canada.[53] If so, it is unfortunate, for in the United States such conflict has led to costly inertia in the health system. The solution lies not in a victory for either professionals or rationalizers, but rather in linking of physicians and administrators in pursuit of common goals.

Such innovative integration is clearly evident in various institutions across North America. First, a popular approach is the matrix model, in which a program administrator, often a doctor, is in charge of a specific type of patient service, such as ophthalmology or digestive diseases. This individual has vertical responsibility for a specific department and horizontal responsibility for coordinating all resources under its program. This decentralized authority, organized around "product lines," enhances liaison between administrators and doctors and is said to result in reduced costs and improved patient care.[54] Second, a more complex variation on the basic matrix combines a traditional administrative structure with not only a programmatic dimension, such as ageing or trauma, but also separate clinical units for specialized areas, such as extended care. Physicians responsible for resource deployment are thus actually aware of and accountable for their expenditures, on the basis of volume and type of cases. Integral participation by doctors in the management process ensures this awareness.[55] Third, another option incorporates them directly into planning, prioritization, and cost-control on a programmatic basis but reserves active program management for advisory committees composed of various health professionals.[56] Fourth, in the United Kingdom the use of clinical directorates became popular during the 1980s. In this approach a clinician is given budgetary control over a hospital subunit and is accountable for resources consumed.[57] Regardless of the approach selected, physicians, by joining management in planning resource deployment, acquire a new awareness of and responsibility for allocative decisions likely to decrease expenditures and increase hospital efficiency. Already, there is evidence that this integration has produced tangible results in many Canadian institutions in the form of increased day-surgery, shorter stays, and concise guidelines on the use of expensive technological resources.

Central to this cooperative process is the need for accurate data at the patient level on costs and outcomes. In Ontario, under a global-budget funding system, there was no administrative need for the generation or analysis of such information. But useful data are now available through the work of a non-profit Canadian organization, the Hospital Medical Records Institute, now renamed as the Canadian Institute for Health Information (CIHI). In 1992 it collected 3.8 million discharge abstracts from 631 member hospitals permitting accurate comparisons over a wide range of diagnoses. A decade earlier it introduced its case-mix groups (CMGs) – a classification based on specific body systems, which grouped diagnoses that would be expected to follow similar clinical courses and required similar resources for their management. In 1987 it added its resource-intensity weights (RIWs), which assign to each CMG a relative quantity of resource consumption, based on Canadian length-of-stay data and modified New York state data on cost per case (comparable Canadian cost figures being as yet unavailable). The weight of 1 (= Can$2,000 in 1991–2), represents the average of resource requirements for all cases in the CIHI database. Thus, for example, a kidney transplant would command an RIW of 5, and care of a normal newborn, 0.22. By using CMGs and RIWs, hospitals can compare the case mix and resource consumption of individual physicians, whole departments, or entire hospitals.[58]

Such comparisons can make physicians aware of costs, which translates into reduced expenditures,[59] and has important implications for the quality of care and the development of treatment guidelines.[60] Some American assessments of the cost impact of the somewhat similar diagnostic related groups (DRGs), however, have been disappointing.[61] As well, Canadian authorities, while recognizing the absence of alternatives, question the validity of using American cost data in the calculation of RIWs.[62] Finally, some observers worry that hospital funding might be adversely affected[63] or directly manipulated by funding authorities[64] through the weights assigned to specific cases. Yet the promise of detailed information on patient-level costs and care cannot be ignored; with such data physicians and administrators in concert will be able to monitor accurately and then alter hospital activities.

Even when supported by accurate data, however, physicians in managerial roles are likely to face several significant difficulties. They usually lack the formal training necessary to approach with confidence highly technical aspects of management, such as accounting. They may be adding administrative duties to an existing clinical role and so perform neither adequately. The introduction of physician managers will threaten organizational structures already in place[65] and, in the case of matrix designs, may fragment lines of authority. Allied health professionals may resent managerial physicians, viewing them as symptoms of a return to medical dominance. By assuming a bureaucratic role, doctors may alienate themselves from former medical colleagues for whom they must now perform auditing and resource-allocation functions. Finally, physicians may find themselves torn between their medical allegiance to individual patients and their institutional loyalty, which demands a potentially different view of cost control and use.[66]

Despite such problems, however, there are clear advantages to integrating doctors into hospital administrations.[67] Physicians have a unique ability to communicate with other physicians, which allows them to recruit colleagues to support administrative goals. For example, by communicating cost awareness and demonstrating the trade-offs dictated by scarce resources, medical managers can help reduce hospital costs through the elimination of inappropriate or inefficient practices. By orchestrating peer review within institutions and sponsoring the development of treatment protocols, they can knowledgeably and with colleagues' support improve patient care. Finally, by joining with hospital bureaucrats to pursue common goals, they can help create the perception that institutional policies are best formulated through a team approach. In time, other groups within the hospital may choose to contribute to this cooperative model.

In testimony to the advantages of integration of physicians into hospital managerial roles, a large number of doctors have sought training and careers in administration.[68] In the United States, six thousand doctors belong to the American College of Physician Executives, and board examinations signify the recognition of management as a specialty. Canada can boast of the success of the

Physician Manager Institute, a joint venture of the CMA and the Canadian College of Health Service Executives.[69] In the United Kingdom, following the report of the National Health Service Management Inquiry in 1983, the British Medical Association formally endorsed the concept of management by physicians.[70] Medical bureaucrats, in short, are part of a wider Anglo-American trend that seeks the more efficient and effective management of the health care system.

The "doctors' workshop," it is clear, faces a critical stage in its evolution. Confronted by costs that must not only be stabilized but also reduced, hospitals have been forced to confront and modify traditional patterns of use. In Ontario, under the close scrutiny since 1995 of the powerful Health Services Restructuring Commission, local institutions will be reconfigured and areas of waste or duplication will be identified for correction. Central to this process are revisions to two outdated and dysfunctional aspects of the physician's activities in hospitals. First, the role of individual hospitals must not be primarily a fortuitous reflection of the interests of its medical staff but rather must represent a clearly articulated attempt to meet the needs of the patient constituency that it serves. Second, the traditional dualism within institutions between physicians and administrators must be bridged through integration of doctors into appropriate management positions.

Admittedly, as the case of revised hospital boards in Quebec during the 1970s suggests,[71] not all changes in hospital structure produce the intended results. Nor do changes at the top of an institution necessary filter down to grass-roots practice, as studies on cost awareness and participation in quality-assurance programs[72] illustrate. But if hospitals are to cope effectively the the pressing issues that confront them – community and long-term care alternatives, proliferation of life-support capacities, evaluation of expensive new technology, and reduction of adverse events, to name but a few – they would do well to begin by restructuring the institutional role of physicians.

6 The Pied Piper of Technology?

Technology is the medical profession's touchstone, a form of tangible substantiation for the physician's claim to pre-eminence within the health care system. But for many professionals, including health economists, policy analysts, and biomedical engineers, the role of technology is far more problematic. Following a brief introduction to the evolution of technology in medicine, this chapter discusses the dilemma posed by technology under three broad headings – specific aspects of medical technology that occasion problems; major constraints on effective action to resolve these concerns; and tentative suggestions as to appropriate policy initiatives for managing technology. Physicians, it will be seen, are both a major part of the problem and an integral part of the solution.

At the beginning of the seventeenth century, in diagnostic technology for example, a physician based his conclusions on the patient's words, his own observations, and, rarely, limited manual examination. It was not until the first half of the nineteenth century that the physical examination became essential to the diagnostic process, and auscultation with Laennec's newly developed stethoscope occupied a central position in the examination. With this rudimentary technology, physicians began the process of peering inside the human body – ironically, to the increasing exclusion of the patient from active participation in the diagnostic exercise.

Ophthalmoscopy, sphygmonamometry, and radiography appeared before the end of the century to further doctors' reliance on implements designed to reveal the pathological secrets of the patient's body. These seemingly primitive instruments were the conceptual forerunners of today's magnetic resonance imaging (MRI) scans or echocardiographs. Despite an assortment of philosophical, economic and clinical reservations, as one scholar has argued, by the late twentieth century "the physician has become a prototype of technological man."[1]

Clinical practice today reveals a bewildering array of medical technology. It includes equipment and instruments, drugs, techniques or procedures, and organizational settings necessary to support the delivery of these resources. The purpose of the technology may be diagnostic, or preventive, or therapeutic, a class that includes curative, rehabilitative, supportive, and palliative therapies. In each such category varying levels of technology are available – high – coronary artery bypass surgery, for example; medium, which includes procedures such as transbronchial biopsy via bronchoscopy; and low, with an example being the routine Pap smear.[2]

Until mid-twentieth century the deployment of medical technology tended to be primarily a private matter between physician and patient rather than an issue of public policy. During the 1960s, if technology entered the policy arena it was largely so that supporters could ensure its rapid proliferation. In the United States, for example, the Regional Medical Program was established in 1965 to push for expeditious adoption of new technologies relevant to heart disease, cancer, and stroke.[3] But medical technology, it gradually became clear, differs in several important ways from other forms of technology. First, there is no real market mechanism for it, since it is usually financed by a third party and the decision to consume is made not by the patient but by the supplying medical practitioner. Second, technology is deployed in industry to achieve cost reductions: in health care, without reference to cost. The ability to document or quantify health outcomes as a consequence of the deployment of a specific technology at a particular cost is all but lacking in clinical practice.[4]

In addition to existing concerns that medical technology has intruded on the human side of the doctor–patient relationship,

economists and epidemiologists worry that technology has under-
gone costly proliferation for poorly documented benefit. Such concerns – about costs, benefits, and the diffusion process – are the
focus for this section of this chapter.

That medical technology is expensive seems obvious from count-
less individual examples. In the United States the cost per successful delivery after one cycle of in vitro fertilization treatment is
$66,667, a figure that rises to $114,286 with the sixth attempt.[5]
Also in obstetrics, to perform amniocentesis and chorionic villus
sampling on all pregnant women in the United States aged 35 and
older would cost $103,329 and $111,184 respectively per abnormal birth averted.[6]

But what do these large dollar figures really mean? First, for a
Canadian audience, they are compromised by their American origin. Ontario, using a centralized provincial source for hospital
funding and a global budget format for each institution, has limited increases in hospital expenditures in general and spending on
technology acquisition in particular.[7] Higher American hospital
costs, in contrast, may be the result of less efficient use of technology – for example, duplication of services by close but competing
hospitals[8] – and application of more services and more expensive
services per admission.[9] Second, bare statements of dollar expenditures do little to gauge the true cost of a technology. One should
obtain estimates of extra costs required to achieve a unit of extra
benefit such as deaths avoided ("cost-effectiveness ratios"), incorporate units that consider the quality of life gained ("cost-utility
ratios"), and translate clinical outcomes into dollar values ("cost-
benefit ratios").[10]

Despite these significant caveats, fragmentary evidence, largely
American, points to technological change as a significant factor in
the increased costs of health care. During the mid-1970s in the
United States, despite relative stability in the total number of tests
and procedures deployed for common diagnoses,[11] there was a significant rise in use of new and more costly diagnostic procedures.[12]
Admittedly, an alternative view attributes the major share of cost
increases to excessive use of "little-ticket" technologies.[13] But
whether one blames CT scanners or inexpensive haemoglobin
determinations, deployment of technology seems a major contrib-
utor to the rising cost of hospital care in particular and of the
health care system in general.[14]

Despite evidence of technology's substantial cost, opinion appears at best divided as to its benefits vis-à-vis health care. Clinicians, by necessity focused on the well-being of individual patients, have few doubts about technology's benefits. Support for such beliefs may indeed be found in the literature, as, for example, in the fact that availability of technology in intensive-care units is significantly associated with lower risk-adjusted mortality.[15] But from a population health perspective the issue is far more problematic. Perhaps the best-known recent exponent of this viewpoint has been Thomas McKeown, who argues persuasively that increased life expectancy in the nineteenth and twentieth centuries owes far more to enhanced nutritional status than to health care.[16]

McKeown's sweeping historical perspective renders his analysis both remote and debatable for physicians. It is possible, however, to focus a critique of technology's role more precisely by examining recent medical practice. There are essentially three arguments. First, recent clinical practice is littered with the remains of ill-conceived technologies and outright medical mistakes. Between 1910 and 1950, for example, thousands of children were irradiated for what was incorrectly considered pathological thymic hyperplasia. The principal result was a significant incidence of radiation-induced cancer of the thyroid as these patients grew to adulthood. Many other examples might be cited – insulin coma for the treatment of schizophrenia, gastric freezing for peptic ulcers, use of diethylstilbesterol and thalidomide during pregnancy – but the message is clear: medical technology may be the author of much serious morbidity or mortality.[17]

A second, less aggressive criticism of technology argues that even seemingly simple and reliable technology may not only fail to do what it claims but may occasion results that are both costly to the system and harmful to the patient. Consider the popular notion that early detection of disease through screening procedures leads to more effective intervention, while a negative test can do no harm. The pap smear is clearly effective in detecting cervical cancer, but it does miss 5 to 20 per cent of cancers on a single screening, while producing false-positive reports in 1 to 10 per cent of cases. The natural course of patients with truly abnormal Pap smears is not always predicable, rendering the cost and effect of follow-up treatment and outcomes difficult to assess precisely. It is known that if all women in the United States were screened every four years from ages twenty to seventy-five the estimated increase in average life expectancy would be approximately three months. The cost of annual screening for this group of patients would be $6 billion, while screening every eligible patient every two years, as is usually recommended, results in a cost of $263,000 per life-year saved. An effective technology introduces questions of frequency of use, cost, accuracy of results, and appropriate follow-up, all of which render its use far more problematic on a population basis than would first appear. The case is even more disturbing for screening tests that lack the Pap smear's effectiveness – that is, clear evidence of effective treatment for the condition sought and proof that early treatment is more effective than late. Two examples from current practice are screening for high cholesterol and examining for prostate cancer.[18] Even simple medical technologies may arguably prove of considerable cost and variable benefit.

A third line of argument as to the role of medical technology, perhaps the most disconcerting, might be styled McKeownism writ small. It examines reductions in morbidity and mortality over a narrow historical period for very specific conditions and particular technological interventions. McKinlay and McKinlay demonstrate that of the total fall in the mortality rate in the United States between 1900 and 1973, over 92 per cent occurred prior to 1950. Paradoxically, the mid-century mark also represents the take-off point for the precipitous increase in the percentage of the American gross national product (GNP) spent on health care. This proportion almost doubled from 1953 to 1973, yet the period accounts for only 8 per cent of the decline in mortality. Focusing on the declining mortality from infectious diseases in the twentieth century, the authors argue that interventions usually were introduced decades after a declining trend had begun and ascribe at most 3.5 per cent of the decline in mortality since 1900 to medical measures.[19]

Broadly similar but more detailed findings come from Bunker, Frazier, and Mosteller. After reviewing screening and immunization procedures in the United States, they concluded that such procedures have added eighteen months to life expectancy when averaged across the whole population. Curative services are more impressive, adding three and a half years. Estimates of the impact of medical intervention on the quality of life are far more difficult to generalize. Cholecystectomy, for example, may bring symptomatic relief to two-thirds of patients with gallbladder disease within two years. Medication for migraine confers pain resolution in up to three-quarters of sufferers. Treatment of high blood pressure reduces the incidence of strokes by half.[20] It is clear from these arguments that medical technology can claim accomplishments, particularity curative and symptomatic, but that there are respectable grounds for believing that its contribution to the population's health may have been exaggerated.

In addition to citing costs and achievements, critics of medical technology focus on a third significant issue – the rapid and uncoordinated manner in which technology is known to diffuse in the health-care sector. McKinlay describes the stages in the evolution of a medical innovation. A promising report based on extremely limited observational evidence is often rapidly embraced by powerful interests in the medical community, which seek both improved patient care and enhanced professional stature. It is a short step to acceptance by professional organizations whose endorsements then create favourable public opinion and lead to formal approval by the state or other sources of third-party funding. To this stage there has been no formal evaluation of the innovation, and even as it assumes the status of a standard procedure assessment takes place largely in the form of retrospective studies or case reports. Only at this belated stage are costly and time-consuming randomized clinical trials initiated and eventually reported. Occasionally they show innovations to be no more effective and perhaps more costly than earlier alternatives, which results elicit denunciation from the innovation's long-time supporters. Gradually, as evidence accumulates and time passes, the innovation is rejected or simply neglected and no longer occasions clinical interest. Clearly some forms of technology may rapidly assume the status of a standard procedure not on the basis of scientific evaluation but rather as a result of physicians' opinions and preferences.[21]

McKinlay's paradigm obviously involves broad generalizations, but the thrust of its argument appears applicable to the diffusion of several recent innovations in medical technology. Consider, for example, the well-documented case of the CT scanner. It was a medical imaging device first introduced to the United States in 1973; four years later there were 401 scanners in that country, compared to twenty-one in Great Britain.[22] By the time the first one hundred devices were installed, only thirteen papers had been published on its principal use – head scanning;[23] though early purchasers cited the favourable cost-benefit ratio of the machines as their second most frequent reason for purchasing units, no such information was then available.[24] Indeed, well into the 1980s it remained unclear whether the technologies that CT scanning wholly or partially displaced – in the case of head scans, arteriography, radionucleotide scans, and pneumoencephalography – were inferior or what the trade-offs in costs were. Nor was this saga of indiscriminate proliferation solely an American experience. In Ontario, despite repeated threats by the provincial government to deny purchase and operating funds to unapproved acquisitions, between 1974 and 1986 the province acquired forty-seven scanners, many purchased without the Ministry of Health's approval.[25]

It would be naïve to assume that this well-publicized case of proliferation has proven a cautionary tale which has curbed physicians' enthusiasm for new imaging technology. Indeed, recent history may repeat itself with MRI scanners. The first image was produced in 1973, and a decade later forty-three scanners were found in the United States, largely in research institutions. In 1984 a report from the (U.S.) Office of Health Technology Assessment was sufficiently positive to motivate the Health Care Financing Administration to issue reimbursement guidelines. Insurers began to pay for MRI scans, and, predictably, by 1993 large numbers of American units (3,647) were in operation, even though their use for purposes beyond the central nervous and musculoskeletal systems was not well established. In fact, only in the early 1990s was MRI scanning subjected to intensive evaluation, and initial results were disappointing.[26] Yet in debt-ridden Ontario, the Ministry of Health announced in late 1994 plans to triple the province's MRI capacity.[27]

How does one explain this seemingly irrational yet endlessly repeated process by which medical technology proliferates and diffuses? The phenomenon is obviously the result of a complex interaction between a variety of factors, including the inherent characteristics of the technology (cost, complexity, purpose), the characteristics of the physicians involved in use of the technology (training, practice formats, payment mechanisms, medical-school affiliations), and the broader health-care environment (financial conditions, government regulations, and malpractice litigation).[28]

Within this complex web of interactions, however, it would appear that the medical profession is the principal force. This pivotal role becomes most clear in the manner in which hospitals – technology's primary location – choose to acquire and use its products. The "key adoption and utilization decisions are in general made by or for physicians,"[29] concluded David Feeny, while Robert Evans writes, "Physicians both determine what procedures are performed in hospitals ... and, what is critically important, constitute the most important pressure group, the 'demand side' of the market, for expansion in facilities."[30] Two studies by Deber and colleagues lend tentative support to these generalizations. In reviewing procedures for technology acquisition first in Ontario[31] and later Canada-wide,[32] they found that doctors initiated many of the requests for new technology, were a major source of information on the value of the recommended technologies, played important roles on committees that approved purchases, and in most institutions were not hampered by any demanding assessment procedures. At least some of these key medical activities, albeit with national idiosyncrasies, appear to be shared by physicians in Britain and the United States.[33] The unrestrained enthusiasm of doctors for medical technology, evident in micro-level studies of hospitals, may well explain the macro-level observations of rapid proliferation made by technology's critics.

Expensive, sometimes of questionable effectiveness, and given to rapid proliferation, medical technology clearly demands some form of regulatory intervention. Yet there are powerful constraints on such action. First, there is a failure of political will to initiate and enforce effective regulation. Second, the medical profession and others are divided as to methods appropriate to the evaluation of technology. Third, past experience suggests that physicians, even when well informed as to the appropriate use of particular technologies, fail to adhere to clinical-usage guidelines. Fourth and finally, physicians' affinity for medical technology is not merely a whim; rather, the need to personify, as a profession, the values represented by science stands at the very core of the medical identity and is not easily circumscribed by external agencies.

In most North American jurisdictions it is clear that the regulation of medical technology carries a low priority on the political agenda. Consider, for example, the three-year career of the National Center for Health Care Technology in the United States.[34] Founded in 1978, in response to concerns over rising costs of medical innovation, its mission was to evaluate the use of existing and emerging technologies in terms of a broad range of factors, including cost, efficacy, and ethics. It was also obliged to provide opinions to Medicare authorities on issues of reimbursement, in which role it saved federal authorities between $100 and $200 million yearly. This appeared a reasonable return from an organization with a budget of barely $4 million annually, and some organizations, such as the American College of Physicians and private insurance companies, gave it considerable support. But they faced more powerful enemies in the American Medical Association, the Health Industry Manufacturers Association, and the competing National Institutes of Health. The centre was accused of stifling technology, limiting physicians' freedom to manage patients, and acting as a federal regulatory agency. These arguments appealed to the free-market views of many members of Congress, and no funds were allocated for operations after 1981.[35] Though some of the centre's duties would be later (1984) bequeathed to the National Center for Health Services Research,[36] politicians in the early 1980s gave in to the vocal enemies of the centre and lacked the resolve to demand a role for technology regulation or assessment.

Canadian politicians have, for the most part, yet to address the issue of technology assessment. British Columbia and Quebec have formally created bodies to advise them on technology evaluation,[37] while all the provinces and the federal government together have sponsored, at a cost of $500,000 in 1991, the Canadian Coordinating office for Health Technology Assessment.[38] But these tentative efforts have little ability to influence practice. In Ontario, as a result, technology appears to proliferate almost randomly. The provincial government divides hospital funds into operational and capital budgets, with expensive new technology purchased with the latter. Such equipment purchases in theory require endorsement from local district health councils as well as the Ministry of Health, so that some degree of restraint and planning is clearly possible. But how does the system respond to technological pressure in practice, particularly for new products that do not represent capital expenditures but are expensive?

The case of low-osmolarity contrast mediums (LOCMs) for radiological procedures is instructive. They became available in Canada in 1986, and their manufacturers promoted them on the grounds of fewer side-effects than traditional contrast mediums. Faced with conversion to a product of as yet unestablished benefit at a cost calculated to increase the health care budget by 0.7 per cent, the Ontario Ministry of Health refused to allocate additional funds. Shortly thereafter, two patients died of allergic reactions to the older mediums, and inquest juries recommended use of LOCMs in future. Hospitals feared liability, on advice from their insurers; physicians learned from their malpractice association that patients should be free to choose LOCM; and the OMA's Section on Radiology urged conversion to the new technology. Though an authoritative British study showed that complete conversion to LOCMs would save only fifteen lives in the United Kingdom yearly, at a cost of U.S.$1 million each, Ontario ignored such considerations. Under public and professional pressure, its government capitulated and made available partial funding for LOCMs without any firm notions of real costs or potential benefits. Other cases, such as the routine use of tissue plasminogen activator for heart-attack victims and the management of asymptomatic elevated cholesterol, show somewhat more resolve on the part of Ontario's government to inhibit the inappropriate proliferation of medical technology.[39] But as the case of LOCMs clearly illustrates, failure of political will is an expensive and not uncommon event vis-à-vis medical innovation.

One likely reason why politicians and bureaucrats may appear ambivalent about technology evaluation – and a second major constraint on effective technology policy – is divided opinion within the medical community itself. Despite its consensus that technology requires thorough evaluation before adoption, particularly through randomized control trials, it has no such agreement on the details of the assessment process. In 1992 a group of Canadian authors, several well-known for previous work in the field,[40] published tentative guidelines for use of clinical and economic analyses to evaluate decisions to adopt or use competing technologies.[41] The result was a brief burst of academic controversy, which revealed just how divided were even those physicians concerned about technology.

The authors of the controversial paper made two basic points. First, they argued that all research on a particular technology should be graded for completeness on a four-point scale, according to whether the study adequately evaluated effectiveness, cost, and impact on quality of life. Second, they devised five grades of recommendation based on the likely magnitude of costs required to achieve additional units of benefit. A grade A recommendation would indicate a technology that was both as effective as and less costly than an existing method, while an E would suggest rejection of a technology that was no more effective than an existing one but also more costly. Combining levels of evidence and grades of recommendation, the authors felt, could result in useful advice on technology deployment. For example, level-one evidence that a technology was in group A would provide compelling justification for its adoption. Throughout their paper the authors conceded that there were a number of limitations to their system such as its arbitrary use of dollar values, the subjective component in quality-adjusted life-years (QALYs), the difficulty associated with rejecting an established technology, the practical problems of incorporating economic considerations into clinical trials, and the mitigating influence of ethical and political factors. Yet they remained convinced that their method offered a rational framework for assessing technologies that would otherwise receive no rigorous evaluation.

The article provoked strong disagreement. Two economists disputed both its main assumptions and its policy implications and provided an alternative method. A new technology, they argued, may prove better than an existing one but is very seldom less expensive. Adopting all such innovations, as the original paper recommended, would therefore inevitably increase the overall cost of health care, unless one assumed the existence of a large and accessible pool of underemployed resources from which to offset new costs. Since cost control is a major motive for technology assessment, the proposed method appeared fatally flawed. Instead, the two economists suggested avoiding QALYs and employing what they considered more objective healthy-years equivalents (HYES) or willingness-to-pay (WTP) measurement. This method, they argued, would provide a yardstick with which to compare all technologies under a given budget. In order to implement a new technology, it would be necessary to show that elimination of an existing program would generate enough revenue for the new proposal while ensuring that the number of HYES lost would be exceeded by those gained.[42]

A somewhat similar but more eclectic critique of the original paper came from a group of Toronto clinicians and epidemiologists. For most technology, they argued, it is impossible to calculate survival gains in person-years precisely because of the absence of long-term data, while quality-of-life estimates will vary with the stage of a disease. Similarly, estimates of cost-effectiveness may vary depending on whether they are derived from a highly specialized setting or from a community venue, and costs will also change from the clinical-trial stage to a time when greater experience may improve efficiency. As a result, a ratio of costs to QALYs will be based on two imprecise factors and may be subject to extraordinary errors. The Toronto group dismissed as outdated and invalid the dollar values used in the original paper, disputed the availability of methods to rank precisely the quality of evidence in studies of technology, and emphasized that a purely utilitarian approach to technology did not necessarily accord with the philosophical or political assumptions underlying Canadian health care.[43]

Many of the issues raised in this debate over the suggested guidelines for technology assessment resuscitated controversies well established in the literature.[44] The present concern is not to determine which view is correct but rather to show that academic debate, though necessary, may inhibit the type of concrete action that would occur if a consensus existed. Until agreement exists on at least an interim form of technology assessment, it will remain unapplied.

Assuming that method is agreed upon, technology assessment is useful primarily in two contexts. First, it may significantly influence initial decisions on acquisition, which in the end are funding decisions taken by government. Second, it may determine appropriate rules for use – an area that is almost entirely medical. The latter implication of assessment in fact constitutes a third major constraint on effective policy towards medical technology. What evidence is there that physicians, when presented with well-conceived guidelines for deployment of a specific technology, will respond appropriately?

The current medical literature reveals at best a divided response on the issue of clinical guidelines. Some recommendations that focus on a very precise issue may influence practice behaviour. Following publication of the results of a major American trial of surgical approaches to breast cancer in 1985, deployment of older surgical techniques declined precipitously in Ontario.[45] Such behaviour change in response to a single publication is doubtless rare, but active educational intervention may prove effective. A study of 120 U.S. hospitals demonstrated an appropriate educational program that could reduce use of x-ray pelvimetry by two-thirds.[46] If direct financial disincentives to hospitals are coupled with physician-generated guidelines, as in the case of the tissue-type plasminogen activator in Ontario, inappropriate application of a specific technology may decline.[47] But alongside these encouraging results are less optimistic examples. Though 78 per cent of Ontario's family physicians surveyed claimed familiarity with guidelines on the appropriate use of cholesterol screening in asymptomatic patients, as few as 5 per cent actually followed the recommendations.[48] Similarly, though the vast majority of obstetricians surveyed were aware of and agreed with a national consensus statement recommending decreased rates of cesarean section, actual practice did not change.[49] Similar disappointing responses to authoritative guidelines have been noted elsewhere,[50] suggesting that persuading physicians to use technology appropriately is a major policy hurdle.

A fourth and final constraint on the formulation of medical-technology policy derives from the nature of the medical profession itself, specifically its self-image. The abstract notion of science, of which some see technology as the concrete application, has long been central to medicine's identity. In the Anglo-American world, long before it possessed the science of effective intervention, the medical profession unconsciously traded on the literate public's growing notion of science as a worthy and respectable body of knowledge. The process had subtle origins in the late eighteenth century. Though bloodied by frequently fatal and always brutal surgery, possessed only of vague theories of humoural pathology, and dispensing often toxic medications, physicians were nonetheless gradually accepted into polite society as representatives of applied science. Recently outsiders little better than tradesmen, physicians had smoothed their passage into middle-class society by deploying not yet the results but the vocabulary of science, a mode of expression that gave a coherent explanatory scheme to the ways of nature, even if it lacked means to intervene in the natural course of disease.

Over the nineteenth century medical science evolved, as did the social authority of the medical profession. In the 1880 the causative organisms were identified for malaria, tuberculosis, cholera, and typhoid. If these diseases lacked a cure, medicine now rid its pharmacopoeia of the worst excesses of heroic therapy and instead deployed therapeutic doses of useful drugs such as digitalis, morphine, and thyroid extract. Surgery, following the introduction of anaesthesia and antiseptic method, became a routine therapy by the 1880s. In parallel with these biomedical innovations, the medical profession organized and delineated its sphere of influence. Lay authorities were displaced in hospitals, medical schools and licensing requirements became increasingly exclusive, and the profession in its journals and societies displayed the organizational attributes of a mature profession.

By 1900 science and medicine were locked in a symbiotic relationship, which the ensuing century would see augmented but largely unchallenged. It was a relationship that provided justification for medicine's privileged social and intellectual status. In fact, medical science, by virtue of its seemingly detached and value-transcendent character, as well as its highly esoteric nature, became inaccessible to lay understanding and largely immune from lay interference.[51] Under such a social paradigm, the notion of exogenous regulation of medical technology became all but an impossibility. Regulation, if it is to succeed, demands the willing participation of physicians themselves.

How then may medical technology be managed? As shown above, medical technology is subject to at least three criticisms – high cost, uncertain benefits, and uncontrolled diffusion. And at least four factors inhibit formulation of policy to redress these worries – lack of resolve on the part of governments, disagreement among physicians on methods of assessing technology, paucity of documentation that evidence-based guidelines on usage will be incorporated into clinical practice, and the fragile self-image of medicine, which will resist external regulation of medical technology. Despite such constraints, however, it is clear that policy initiatives are both necessary and, at least in a preliminary sense, feasible. Suggestions here focus on four distinct elements – individual physicians, hospitals, regional authorities, and a proposed national coordinating body.

An effective approach to technology management must build into the system at a basic level, a conceptual "buy-in" by physicians. The medical profession is instrumental in the development, diffusion, and deployment of technology; if it lacks respect for the tenets of appropriate assessment and use, its members will continue to create rather than solve technology problems. Inculcating such beliefs must start in medical school, not simply as a segment of a single course but as a facet of every clinical lecture dealing with the diagnostic and therapeutic management of patients. Such learning must become a routine component of continuing medical education and must be reinforced by published guidelines on uses. Only by making this fundamental commitment to fully informed decisions on use, will physicians be able to counter credibly the accusation made by authoritative economists[52] and policy analysts[53] that inappropriate medical decision-making is the fundamental problem in management of medicine technology.

The efficacy of educational interventions, particularly for practicing physicians, is problematic,[54] but such actions may be buttressed with other policy choices aimed directly at modifying clinical behaviour. Use of technology has long been known to correlate with the educational background and specialty of physicians.[55] First, manpower planning designed to alter the ratio of specialists to family physicians might influence the use of technology. Second, practice format has been shown to affect use of health care resources. The rate of hospitalization in American health maintenance organizations (HMOs)[56] and in Ontario health service organizations(HSOs)[57] is lower than it is in fee-for-service practice. This finding suggests that rostered patients consume less hospital-based medical technology. Third, remuneration of physicians could be altered so as to discourage unwelcome enthusiasm for technology. Under the current fee-for-service system, which often favours procedure-oriented practice, there are no incentives for physicians either to use technology appropriately or to educate patients in the appropriate use of health care resources. Various modifications to the reimbursement system, including new concepts such as "interim fees," which could be billed only by those physicians participating in the introductory studies of a new technology[58] or sessional payments, which would replace volume-driven fees and have been introduced in some of Ontario's academic centres, might restrain the hasty adaptation of many technologies.

If physicians must be recruited to the cause of appropriate deployment of technology, so too must hospitals. There are a number of policy options open to the Ministry of Health to encourage such compliance. First, though completely ignored by a recent review committee,[59] revision of the Public Hospitals Act should make an exacting and uniform process of intra-institutional technology assessment a mandatory prerequisite to technology acquisition above a certain dollar value for both purchase and yearly operation. Second, if physicians are incorporated into the bureaucratic structure of the hospital, as suggested above in chapter 5, they could devise and enforce evidence-based guidelines for use of hospital technologies. Third, other funding options might supplement the global budget format for hospitals used during the 1970s and 1980s, which proved reasonably appropriate for curbing capital expenditures and might, even in modified form, be continued. The experience of several American jurisdictions with prospective payment plans, for example, suggests that carefully designed programs may curb technology proliferation.[60] Fourth and finally, a more radical policy departure envisages controlling technology costs by deliberately shifting delivery of services to non-institutional settings, enhancing the facilities available for self-care, and recruiting service provision by less costly and less highly trained personnel.[61] Already there is clear evidence that hospital administrators strongly agree that new technologies must be evaluated. [62] Taken together, the above policy options offer effective measures to permit control of technology deployment in hospitals.

Beyond institutions, there is clearly a role in technology control for the increasingly popular concept of regional devolution. This notion anticipates "envelope funding" from the province and, though the one major report on regionalization made no mention of it,[63] could incorporate mandatory provisions for technology acquisition. This approach would permit the coordination of technology deployment among regions, perhaps, by way of example, incorporating the type of competitive arrangements foreseen for an "internal market" in Britain's National Health Service.[64] It would also allow regions to "prioritize" within their own boundaries the provision of specialized facilities and to audit more accurately on a manageable scale the use and cost of various technologies. Accompanying provisions for medical personnel planning and for alternative remuneration schemes would also allow regions to influence use of technology. Program budgeting on a region-wide basis would enhance the ability of physicians and administrators to control use of technology according to predetermined guidelines.[65] Regions might be given the ability to exclude completely a given technology, even to the point of relegating it to a free-market setting or insisting that certain marginal technologies carry with them a co-payment provision. Regional devolution, in summary, offers both an opportunity to exert innovative local control over technology and the welcome prospect of fostering a less adversarial relationship between communities and the provincial government.

The final level of policy initiation moves beyond regions and provinces to demand a national effort. To date Canadian attempts to deal with technology, though laudable when compared to many other jurisdictions,[66] have been fragmentary and concerned largely with control through funding mechanisms. This situation has led to demands for a national technology-assessment body to organize domestic evaluations and adapt off-shore data,[67] while simultaneously carefully avoiding an overtly regulatory function. Similar suggestions have been made in the United States, where such an agency might identify current and new technologies requiring evaluation, sponsor evaluations, synthesize existing data, and disseminate the results of the evaluation process to a relevant audience.[68] Necessarily, assessment of any technology incorporates a wide range of concerns, including technical performance, clinical efficacy, safety, cost and efficiency, acceptability to providers and patients, research value, effects on the health care system in organizational terms, and ethical-social issues.[69] While technology assessment faces obvious obstacles, including inherent expense and problems of ensuring that findings are incorporated into clinical practice,[70] it nonetheless is a task best suited to a national government.

It will now be clear that, as was suggested at the beginning of this chapter, physicians are both a cause of the technology problem and a key to its solution. They bear considerable responsibility for past introduction of costly and often poorly evaluated technologies, some later found to be either harmful or useless. If pursuit of status or income helped motivate these actions, there is little evidence to suggest that a sincere desire to enhance health care was not the principal intention. It is this altruistic urge, in fact, that may now provide the motivational springboard from which doctors may leap beyond traditional, neglectful approaches to regulation of technology and help to devise a rational approach to adoption and use. This chapter has described some of the constraints on such policy – lack of political will, confusion over methods of assessment and dissemination of guidelines, and a perceived threat to medical autonomy. But by focusing first on the individual physician and then moving beyond to hospitals, regions, and finally the national level, it has shown how the threat of accelerating costs, questionable benefits, and uncontrolled proliferation may gradually become a policy dilemma of the past.

Conclusion

The year following the buffoonery of the Burlington physician described in the introduction was not a pleasant one for Ontario's minister of health. In the midst of a bitter dispute with physicians, complete with the selective withdrawal of medical services, he was forced to step aside by the public indiscretions of an aide. Months later, after he was exonerated and reinstated in his post, his return to the legislature was blighted by a most unusual event. An opposition member sponsored a resolution condemning the Conservative government's health policy, normally a relatively innocuous parliamentary tactic. On this occasion, however, six government back-benchers broke party ranks to side with the opposition, resulting in a tie vote. Possibly for only the second time in Ontario history, the Speaker, a Tory, was called on to cast the tie-breaking vote, which he did in support of the opposition's condemnatory motion.[1] Like the antics of the Burlington doctor, the vote had little intrinsic significance. Rather, it symbolized the continued discord and disorganization in Ontario's health policy.

By 1997 enthusiasm for community health organizations (CHOs) appeared evanescent, and the brave hopes for rapid regionalization, so evident in the Orser Report in 1991,[2] had apparently been cast aside. Not that such notions were explicitly rejected. Rather, they had been transmuted into a new term, "integrated health systems,"[3] which might be broadly described as an organization or network that provides a coordinated range of services to a defined population and is held responsible, clinically and financially, for the health outcomes for those served.[4] Once again, it seems, the disorganized, uncoordinated status quo would be pitted against a new model of planned health services. The question remains, however, how to transform the present into this structured future and particularly, for purposes of this book, how this transformation might deal with the physician-related policy issues discussed in preceding chapters. To this end, this chapter outlines three major goals and proposes five possible short-term adjustments.

The objective of Ontario's system of health care delivery is to enhance the health status of all citizens. To do so demands that three distinct though related goals be pursued – equity, efficiency, and effectiveness (Table C1). First, concerning equity, acceptable primary and advanced care, including health technology, must be available to all citizens, regardless of gender, age, affluence, and other such criteria. Under the present system, availability of acceptable care is variable, while under a managed system it would be present as a result of needs-based planning. At the same time, providers must be sufficiently satisfied with the equity of the system to work harmoniously within it. At present, there is dissent from physicians, though two-thirds of them are reasonably satisfied with the conditions of practice. A managed system would probably command equal satisfaction from primary-care physicians and greater acceptance over time from the entire profession. This result would be particularily likely in settings such as hospitals where physicians were permitted to assume significant administrative authority.

There is obviously no guarantee that physicians would prefer a managed system. Although half of those surveyed by the Canadian Medical Association in 1995 indicated preference for a payment format other than fee for service, a majority were critical of and felt excluded by regionalization programs in their areas. Yet only 15 per cent of respondents found the status quo "very acceptable," suggesting openness to reasonable alternatives.[5] An integrated system offers a number of advantages that speak to the two primary concerns of most physicians – appropriate remuneration and optimal patient care. A devolved system offers practitioners the opportunity to exert greater influence within the local practice environ-

Table C1
Goals and results in current and managed systems

Goals*	Evaluation criteria	Results	
		Current system	Managed system
Equity	Acceptable care avail-able to all residents	Unpredictable	Needs-based
	Providers satisfied with system	Two thirds satisfied	Probably equal and greater over time
Efficiency	Accessibility high	Distribution dis–parities	Disparities reduced
	Cost predictable and appropriate	Growth curtailed and predictable within limits	Predictable
	Physicians integrated into management	Slight	Increased
Effectiveness	Necessary diagnostic and treatment inter-ventions undertaken	Little deprivation or queuing	Equal
	Unnecessary diagnostic and treatment inter-ventions not under-taken	Considerable over servicing	Greatly reduced
	Appropriate evaluation of medical technology	No incentives	Enhanced incentives

*Objective: Improved health for Ontario residents.

ment in contrast to a centralized system. They would have more say in what resources the community should acquire and subsequent access to those resources. Patient care could be better coordinated in smaller regions that control their own allocative decisions. Some of the cost savings associated with more efficient organization might reasonably be passed on to physicians as incentives for providing appropriate and effective patient care. Alternates to the status quo, in short, hold both altruistic and entrepreneurial attractions to doctors.

The second goal of the system must be efficiency. Medical care must be accessible to all citizens, and costs must be both predictable and appropriate. At present there are regional disparities

Table C2
Five policy variables in transitional and managed systems

Policy variables and chapter where discussed	Transitional system	Managed system
Remuneration (Chapter 2)	OHIP aggregate payout capped; individual caps in place for specialists and general practitioners Non-essential services removed from OHIP benefits Abuse of OHIP by commercial house-call services and walk-in clinics forbidden	Capitation for family physicians; sessional contracts for specialists
Supply and distribution of physicians (Chapter3)	Undergraduate and postgraduate enrolments reduced Licensing of graduates of foreign medical schools restricted Differential fees in place for new doctors in over and under-serviced areas Enhanced practice incentives in rural areas Hospital privileges restricted in over-serviced areas	Local-generated, needs-based physician resource policy
Quality assessment and assurance (Chapter 4)	OHIP audit and feedback enhanced Under- and postgraduate Q.A. instruction introduced CPSO Peer Review Program expanded Patients educated to demand appropriate care Use of practice guidelines encouraged	Quality assurance programs linked directly to needs-based planning and physicians' remuneration
Institutional management (Chapter 5)	Physicians integrated into management structure Accurate patient-level use data generated Cost awareness among medical staff enhanced	Designated planning and management role for physicians

Table C2 (continued)

Policy variables and chapter where discussed	Transitional system	Managed system
Technology diffusion (Chapter 6)	Extensive physician education on cost and benefits of specific technolgies Mandatory province-wide protocols on hospitals' technology acquisition Regional and inter-regional technology planning through district health councils Contribution to national technology assessment program	Coordinated intra- and inter-regional technology acquisition and use

in the distribution of physicians, which the needs-based planning of a managed system would correct. The cost of physicians' services has been curtailed and rendered somewhat predictable by the capping process added to the current system. The combination of "envelope funding" and planning authority envisaged for devolved authorities would make the prediction and allocation of expenditures on physicians' services far more exact and equitable. A system of managed technology acquisition and use would substantially diminish current cost concerns for unregulated proliferation of technology.

The third goal of the system is effectiveness – patients should receive necessary diagnostic and treatment interventions. At present there is little if any deprivation in an absolute sense and, except in some surgical procedures, relatively little queuing. A managed system would display a similar ability to gratify legitimate medical needs. Of equal importance, however, it would prevent unnecessary diagnostic and treatment interventions – a process in which technology assessment and regulation would play an important role. There is at present considerable overservicing, which managed systems would avoid by severing the link between remuneration and volume of service delivery.

It is clear from the above discussion that the goals of equity, efficiency, and effectiveness are best served by a managed system of health care rather than the present system. Yet none of the three principal stakeholders – government, patients and providers – is likely to welcome abrupt or radical changes. Instead, the current system should be modified by introduction of effective short-term adjustments in the five policy variables discussed in this book – remuneration (chapter 2), physician supply (chapter 3), quality assurance (chapter 4), institutional authority (chapter 5), and technology diffusion (chapter 6) – to provide the basis for a transitional stage on the way to a more managed system (Table C2).

First, a modified version of the current system should deal with physicians' remuneration in new ways, most of which have been very recently initiated or are anticipated. The aggregate OHIP payment to doctors should be subjected to a negotiated cap, and all physicians should have caps placed on their earnings according to their specialty. Non-essential items should be removed from the OHIP schedule, and services that abuse the intention of OHIP, such as commercial house-call services and walk-in clinics, should be prohibited. These changes would significantly inhibit the unbridled entrepreneurialism that characterized Ontario medicine until the mid-1980s. More important, such controlled remuneration would significantly shorten the step to a managed system based on capitated primary care and sessional fees for specialists.

Second, the current system should be adjusted to correct for both an oversupply and a maldistribution of physicians. This may be done by reducing the number of undergraduate and postgraduate training positions, restricting the licensing of graduates of foreign medical schools, enhancing practice conditions in underserviced areas, restricting physicians' access to medical facilities such as hospitals in overserviced areas, and, finally, introducing differential fees to reward appropriate practice locations and deter inappropriate locations. These changes, particularly the link between remuneration and practice location, would ease the transition to a more highly planned structure. A managed system, by relying on needs-based planning, would remove the serendipity that now characterizes distribution of practitioners and would refuse to employ physicians surplus to documented population requirements.

Third, the current system should be modified to enhance quality assessment and assurance. Detailed consideration of this issue must be incorporated into undergraduate and postgraduate training programs, as well as into continuing medical education. The public too must be educated to demand care of appropriate quality. The Ontario Medical Association and other groups should be assisted to introduce and monitor use of clinical practice guidelines. The College of Physicians and Surgeons of Ontario should be assisted in expanding the size and scope of its peer review program as well as its remedial component. By making physicians aware that the state has a legitimate duty to ensure the quality of the care that it purchases, such efforts would pave the way for the more extensive quality-assurance programs likely to result from both integrated delivery systems and regional authorities.

Fourth, hospital administrations should integrate physicians into management at both the program and the institutional levels. This integration would not only allow physicians to participate in the planning of hospital programs and restructuring but would also require them to take responsibility for decisions on resource allocation. Improved data on patient-level use of resources would be essential for such activities and could be employed to foster cost-awareness and behavioural change in all members of the medical staff. Under a managed system of care, such as is represented by current notions of regional devolution, doctors would be expected to participate, along with other stakeholders, in the planning and operation of the region's health care system.

Fifth and finally, the system can clearly take a far more active role in the regulation of technology. For a start, physicians – the group most responsible for introduction and use of new technology – should be educated as to the costs and benefits of competing diagnostic and therapeutic modalities. Institutions should foster a similar awareness by demanding adherence to province-wide protocols for technology acquisition. Effective intra- and inter- regional policies on technology deployment should become a priority for district health councils.The province should make a permanent commitment to cooperate in a national program of technology assessment. As they become more aware that technology brings costs as well as benefits and that deployment must be planned rather that random, physicians will become cognizant of the type of assumptions that underlie the approach taken to technology under a managed care system.

Thus the present health care system, with appropriate modifications, can become not the foil of but a transitional stage to a managed system (see Table C2). This is not only a wise implementation tactic but an absolute prerequisite for adequate evaluation of proposals for future systems. Consider, for example, the growing interest in the popular panacea of devolution. Though already adopted in most provinces, the concept of regional health authorities appears to have a variety of meanings, and its strengths and weaknesses are not well documented. Regional devolution is said by its supporters to have a number of advantages – better representation of community needs and preferences, increased probability of innovative solutions to local health problems, enhanced ability to integrate and coordinate regional health services, and more fiscally responsible deployment of resources through better matching of services to local needs. Critics argue that there are significant problems with the model – appropriate regional boundaries are difficult to define, regional authorities would be more susceptible to political influence and possessed of less technical expertise, uniform provincial standards would be difficult to ensure, contiguous regions might duplicate services rather than cooperate, and regional authorities constitute another level of health bureaucracy.

To date a definitive resolution to these competing views does not exist. Existing studies question the ability of regions to integrate services[6] or to represent local viewpoints fully, while also suggesting that the governance structures in place meet the provincial government's expectations[7] and possess the potential to make a more efficient and dynamic use of health information for planning and delivering services.[8] Perhaps diconcertingly, it has been noted that the regionalization trend in Canada is similar to the type of system that Sweden is beginning to abandon.[9] The point remains, however, that modifying the current system in the short term is preferrable to adopting an entirely new system, which has yet to be adequately evaluated.

Where then does this situation leave physicians? As C.D. Naylor has persuasively argued in his study of physicians and the politics of medicine, a priority for Canadian medicine throughout the century has been maintenance of a practice pattern in which most doctors were self-employed providers operating on a fee-for-service basis. In retrospect, it is clear that building medicare around the existing fee-for-service system guaranteed continued professional independence into the 1980s.[10] The present study has argued that this traditional independence is about to end, the victim of flawed assumptions made by medicare's founders the consequences of which became fully apparent only under the fiscal crisis of the late 1980s. The challenge now is two-fold: first, physicians must accept the inevitability of change and work with the system's managers to achieve an optimal outcome, and second, politicians and bureaucrats must recognize the wealth of expertise that physicians can contribute not just on clinical issues but also on topics such as hospital management and technology assessment. In short, the culture of confrontation that has defined physician–government relations in Ontario for the last two decades should give way to a new model – a construct that abandons the anomaly of private practice and public payment for a truly integrated health system.

Notes

INTRODUCTION

1 "Premier Needs Head Examined, Doc Says," *Kingston Whig-Standard,* 17 Jan., 1996, A1 (Col. 1).
2 S.E.D. Shortt, "Physicians, Science and Status: Issues in the Professionalization of Anglo-American Medicine in the Nineteenth Century," *Medical History,* 27 (1983), 51–68.
3 S.E.D. Shortt, "'Before the Age of Miracles': The Rise, Fall and Rebirth of General Practice in Canada, 1890–1940," in Charles Roland, ed.,Charles Roland, ed., *Health, Disease and Medicine: Essays in Canadian History* (Toronto: Hannah Institute for the History of Medicine, 1984), 123–52.
4 Bernard Blishen, *Doctors in Canada: The Changing World of Medical Practice* (Toronto: University of Toronto Press in association with Statistics Canada, 1991); David Coburn, George Torrance, and Joseph M. Kaufert, "Medical Dominance in Canada in Historical Perspective: The Rise and Fall of Medicine?" *International Journal of Health Services,* 13 (1983); 407–32; Michael Wahn, "The Decline of Medical Dominance in Hospitals," in *Health and Canadian Society, Sociological Perspectives,* 2nd ed., David Coburn, Carl D'Arcy, George Torrence, and Peter New, eds., (Toronto: Fitzhenry and Whiteside, 1987), 422–40.
5 Paul Starr, *The Social Transformation of American Medicine* (New York: Basic Books, 1982).

6 Robin F. Badgley and Samuel Wolfe, *Doctors' Strike, Medical Care and Conflict in Saskatchewan* (Toronto: Macmillan of Canada, 1967).

7 C.D. Naylor, *Private Practice, Public Payment: Canadian Medicine and the Politics of Health Insurance, 1911–1966* (Montreal: McGill-Queen's University Press, 1986), 250.

8 J. Henry, "Policy Written on the Back of a Matchbox," *Ontario Medical Review*, 60 (1993), 1.

9 R.L. Kravitz, L.S. Linn, and M.F. Shapiro, "Physician Satisfaction under the Ontario Health Insurance Plan," *Medical Care*, 28 (1990); 502–512; Diana Swift, ed., *The Medical Post 1992 National Survey of Canadian Doctors* (Toronto: Maclean Hunter, 1992).

10 Eliot Freidsen, *Profession of Medicine: A Study of the Sociology of Applied Knowledge* (New York: Harper and Row, 1970), 82.

11 Christel A.Woodward, et al., "When Is a Patient's Use of Primary Care Services Unwarranted? Some Answers from Physicians," *Canadian Medical Association Journal (CMAJ)*, 129 (1983); 822–7; M. Oreilly, "Don't Seek Medical Help for Minor Problems Ontario Pilot Project Tells Patients," *CMAJ*, 15 (1994); 201–2.

12 Roberta Labelle, Greg Stoddard, and Thomas Rice, "A Re-examination of the Meaning and Importance of Supplier-Induced Demand," McMaster University, Centre for Health Economics and Policy Analysis, Working Paper 93–2, Hamilton, 1993.

13 P. Paul-Shaheen, J.D. Clark, and D. Williams, "Small Area Analysis: A Review and Analysis of North American literature," *Journal of Health Politics, Policy and Law*, 12 (1987); 741–805.

14 Sir Douglas Black et al., *Inequalities in Health: The Black Report*, ed. P. Townsend and N. Davidson (Harmondsworth: Penguin Books, 1982).

15 Marianne Lamb et al., *Managed Care in Canada: The Toronto Hospital's Proposed Comprehensive Health Organization* (Ottawa: Canadian Hospital Association Press, 1991).

16 College of Family Physicians of Canada, *Managing Change: The Family Medicine Group Practice Model* (Toronto: College, 1995).

17 Canadian Medical Association, *Core and Comprehensive Health Care Services. A Framework for Decision-making* (Ottawa: Association, 1994).

18 National Ad Hoc Working Group on Physician Resource Planning, *Report of the National Ad Hoc Working Group on Physician Resource Planning* (Ottawa: Working Group, 1995).

19 National Forum on Health, *The Public and Private Financing of Canada's Health System* (Ottawa: Forum, 1995).

20 R. Williams and B. LeBlanc, 'Examining the Workings of the Health Services Restructuring Committee,' *Ontario Medical Review*, 64 (1997); 18–22.

CHAPTER ONE

1 J.J. Rouleau et al., "A Comparison of Management Patterns after Acute Myocardial Infarction in Canada and the United States," *New England Journal of Medicine (NEJM)*, 328 (1993); 779–84.
2 Daniel Mark et al., "Use of Medical Resources and Quality of Life after Acute Myocardial Infarction in Canada and the United States," *NEJM*, 331 (1994); 1130–35.
3 Geoffrey M. Anderson, Joseph P. Newhouse, and Leslie L. Roos, "Hospital Care for Elderly Patients with Diseases of the Circulatory System, A Comparison of Hospital Use in the United States and Canada," *NEJM*, 321 (1989); 1443–8.
4 Geoffrey Anderson et al., "Use of Coronary Artery Bypass Surgery in the United States and Canada, Influence of Age and Income. *Journal of the American Medical Association (JAMA)*, 269 (1993); 1661–9.
5 Leslie L. Roos et al.,"Postsurgical Mortality in Manitoba and New England," *JAMA*, 263 (1990); 2453–8.
6 Peter Coyte et al., "Waiting Time for Knee-replacement Surgery in the United States and Ontario," *NEJM*, 331 (1994); 1063–71.
7 S. Katz, L. McMahon, and W. Manning, "Comparing the Use of Diagnostic Tests in Canadian and U.S. Hospitals," *Medical Care*, 34 (1996); 117–25.
8 Ronald Kessler et al., "Differences in the Use of Psychiatric Outpatient Services between the United States and Ontario," *NEJM*, 336 (1997); 551–7.
9 Steffie Woolhandler and David Himmelstein, "The Deteriorating Administrative Efficiency of the U.S. Health Care System," *NEJM*, 324 (1991); 1253–7.
10 R.J. Blendon et al., "Satisfaction with Health Systems in Ten Nations," *Health Affairs*, 9 (1990); 185–92.
11 J. Chidley, "Radical Surgery, Cuts in Public Funding Imperil Medicare's Future," *Maclean's*, 109 (2 Dec. 1996); 44–7.
12 Ontario Medical Association, "Physician Survey on Health-Care Reform," *Ontario Medical Review*, 62 (1995); 22–9.
13 R.L. Kravitz, L.S. Linn, and M.F. Shapiro, "Physician Satisfaction

under the Ontario Health Insurance Plan," *Medical Care*, 28 (1990); 502–12.

14 R.J. Blendon et al., "Physicians' Perspectives on Caring for Patients in the United States, Canada, and West Germany," *NEJM*, 328 (1993); 1011–16.

15 Government of Ontario. Ministry of Health. "Managing Health Care Resources, Meeting Ontario's Priorities." Supplementary Paper, 1992 Budget. Toronto, 1992.

16 J.C. Stick, "Critical Limits to Taxation," *Canadian Tax Journal*, 40 (1992); 1315–31.

17 C. Nair and R. Karim, "An Overview of Health Care Systems: Canada and Selected OECD Countries," *Health Reports*, 5 (1993); 259–79.

18 Jonathan Lomas, "Finding Audiences, Changing Beliefs: The Structure of Research Use in Canadian Health Policy," *Journal of Health Politics, Policy and Law*, 15 (1990): 525–42.

19 Joan P. Boase, *Shifting Sands, Government–Group Relationships in the Health Care Sector*, (Montreal: McGill-Queen's University Press, 1994).

20 Douglas Angus, *Review of Significant Health Care Commissions and Task Forces in Canada since 1983–84* (Ottawa: Canadian Hospital Association, Canadian Medical Association, Canadian Nurses Association, 1991).

21 Jeremiah Hurley, Jonathan Lomas, and Vanda Bhatia, "Is the Wolf Finally at the Door? Provincial Reform to Manage Health-care Resources," McMaster University, Centre for Health Economics and Policy Analysis, Working Paper 93–12, Hamilton, 1993.

22 D. Chernichovsky, "Health System Reform in Industrialized Democracies: An Emerging Paradigm," *Millbank Quarterly*, 73 (1995); 339–72.

23 S.B. Sheps, Greg Anderson, and Karen Cardiff, "Utilization Management: A Literature Review for Canadian Health Care Administrators," *Healthcare Management Forum*, 4 (1991); 34–9.

24 T.M. Wickizer, "The Effect of Utilization Review on Hospital Use and Expenditures: A Review of the Literature and an Update on Recent Findings," *Medical Care Review*, 47 (1990); 327–63.

25 Greg Anderson, S.B. Sheps, and Karen Cardiff, "Hospital-Based Utilization Management: A Cross-Canada Survey," *Canadian Medical Association Journal (CMAJ)*, 143 (1990); 1025–30.

26 Paula Blackstien-Hirsch, Antoni Basinski, and C.D. Naylor, "Management of Hospital Bed Utilization in Canada–Current Activities and

Potential Strategies," Institute for Clinical Evaluative Sciences in Ontario, Working Paper 10, June 1993.

27 Working Group on Health Services Utilization, "When Less Is Better: Using Canada's Hospitals Efficiently," paper prepared for the Conference of Federal, Provincial, Territorial Deputy Ministers of Health, June 1994.

28 F.P. Harrison, D. Juzwishin, and R. Roger, "Quality of Care and Utilization Management: Contemporary Tools and Strategies," *Healthcare Management Forum*, 2 (1989); 18–23.

29 F.P. Harrison and W.F. Roger, "Quality Utilization Management: Preliminary Results to a Canadian Approach," *Healthcare Management Forum*, 3 (1990); 28–33.

30 Donald M. Berwick, "Health Services Research and Quality of Care, Assignments for the 1990s," *Medical Care*, 27 (1989); 763–71.

31 Donald M. Berwick and Marian G. Knapp, "Theory and Practice for Measuring Health Care Quality," *Health Care Financing Review* (annual supplement, 1987); 49–55.

32 Peter Coyte, D.N. Dewees, and M.J. Trebilcock, "Medical Malpractice: The Canadian Experience," *NEJM*, 324 (1991); 89–93.

33 B.S. Hulka et al., "Peer Review in Ambulatory Care: Use of Explicit Criteria and Implicit Judgments," *Medical Care* (supplement) 17 (1979); 1–65.

34 Health Services Research Group, "Small-Area Variations: What Are They and What Do They Mean?," *CMAJ*, 146 (1992); 467–70.

35 Catherine Fooks, Michael Rachlis, and Carol Kushner, "Assessing Concepts of Quality of Care: Results of a National Survey of Five Self-Regulating Health Professions in Canada," McMaster University, Centre for Health Economics and Policy Analysis, Working Paper 90–7, Hamilton, 1990.

36 J.Casanova, "Status of Quality Assurance Programs in American Hospitals," *Medical Care*, 28 (1990); 1104–9.

37 Government of Ontario, Ministry of Health, Public Hospitals Act Review, *Into the 21st Century, Ontario Public Hospitals*, Report of the Steering Committee, (Toronto, 1992).

38 Kathleen N. Lohr, "Outcome Measurements: Concepts and Questions," *Inquiry*, 25 (1988); 37–50.

39. A.R. Tarlov et al.,"The Medical Outcomes Study; An Application of Methods for Monitoring the Results of Medical Care," *JAMA*, 262 (1989); 925–30.

40 John Wennberg, "Outcomes Research, Cost Containment, and the Fear of Health Care Rationing," *NEJM*, 323 (1990); 1202–4.

41 Health Services Research Group, "Outcomes and the Management of Health Care," *CMAJ*, 147 (1992); 1775–80.

42 Alan Detsky and I.G. Naglie, "A Clinician's Guide to Cost-effectiveness Analysis," *Annals of Internal Medicine*, 113 (1990); 147–54.

43 Stephen Birch and John Eyles, "Needs-Based Planning of Health Care: A Critical Appraisal of the Literature," McMaster University, Centre for Health Economics and Policy Analysis, Working Paper 91–5, Hamilton, 1991.

44 John Eyles and Stephen Birch, "A Population Needs-based Approach to Health-care Resource Allocation and Planning in Ontario: A Link between Policy Goals and Practice?" *Canadian Journal of Public Health*, 84 (1993); 112–17.

45 Stephen Birch and S. Chambers, "To Each According to Need: A Community-based Approach to Allocating Health Care Resources," *CMAJ*, 149 (1993); 607–12.

46 R. Pampalon et al., "The Selection of Needs Indicators for Regional Resource Allocation in the Fields of Health and Social Services in Quebec," *Social Science and Medicine*, 42 (1996); 909–21.

47 Kevin Brazil and Malcolm Anderson, "Assessing Health Service Needs: Tools for Health Planning," *Healthcare Management Forum*, 9 (1996); 22–7; Nina Bullen, Graham Moon, and Kelvyn Jones, "Defining Localities for Health Planning: A GIS Approach," *Social Science and Medicine*, 42 (1996); 801–16.

48 Government of Ontario, Premier's Council on Health Strategy, Report of the Integration and Coordination Committee, *Local Decision Making For Health and Social Services* (Toronto, 1991), 14.

49 John Eyles, "The Role of the Citizen in Health-care Decision-making," McMaster University, Centre for Health Economics and Policy Analysis, Policy Commentary 93–4, Hamilton, 1993.

50 Julie Abelson et al., "Does the Community Want Devolved Authority? Results From Deliberative Polling in Ontario," McMaster University, Centre for Health Economics and Policy Analysis, Working Paper 94–19, Hamilton, 1994.

51 Government of Canada, National Health and Welfare, *Planning for Health: Towards Informed Decision Making* Report of the Project Team on Emerging Trends in the Organization and Delivery of Health Care Services (Ottawa, 1993).

52 Government of Ontario, Ministry of Health, "Goals and Strategic Priorities, Ministry of Health," Working Document (Toronto, 1992).

CHAPTER TWO

1 United States Congress, House, Committee on Government Operations, *Canadian Health Insurance: Lessons for the United States*, GAO/HRD-91–90, June 1991.
2 Edward Neuschler, *Canadian Health Care: The Implications of Public Health Insurance*, Research Bulletin of the Health Insurance Association of America (Boston: 1990).
3 Theodore R. Marmor, "Commentary on 'Canadian Health Insurance: Lessons for the United States,'" Testimony before the House Committee on Government Operations, United States Congress, Washington, DC, 18 June 1991.
4 Government of Ontario, *Managing Health Care Resources: Meeting Ontario's Priorities*, Supplementary Paper, 1992 Ontario Budget (Toronto,1992), 1.
5 Government of Canada, Department of Finance, *Federal–Provincial Study on the Cost of Government and Expenditure Management* (Ottawa, 1992).
6 Ben Chan and Geoffrey Anderson, "Trends in Physician Fee-For-Service Billing Patterns," in Vivek Goel et al., eds., *Patterns of Health Care in Ontario: The ICES Practice Atlas*, 2nd ed. (Ottawa: Canadian Medical Association, 1996).
7 Robert G. Evans, "Health Care in Canada: Patterns of Funding and Regulation," *Journal of Health Politics, Policy and Law*, 8 (1983), 1–43.
8 Allan S. Detsky, Sidney R. Stacey, and Claire Bombardier, "The Effectiveness of a Regulatory Strategy in Containing Hospital Costs," *New England Journal of Medicine (NEJM)*, 309 (1983), 151–9; Allan S. Detsky et al., "Containing Ontario's Hospital Costs under Universal Insurance in the 1980's: What Was the Record?" *Canadian Medical Association Journal (CMAJ)*, 142 (1990),565–72.
9 Ontario Ministry of Health, Health Insurance Division, *Submission to the Task Force on the Use and Provision of Medical Services* (Toronto, Feb. 1990).
10 Darrel Weinkauf and Adam Linton, "Physician Payment in Canada" (letter), *Health Affairs*, 8 (1989), 235–8.
11 Ontario Ministry of Health, *Submission to the Task Force*.

12 Data supplied to the author by the OMA based on OHIP figures.
13 Ontario, *Managing Health Care Resources*, 1.
14 H. Michael Stevenson, A. Paul Williams, and Eugene Vayda, "Medical Politics and Canadian Medicare: Professional Response to the Canada Health Act," *Milbank Quarterly*, 66 (1988), 65–104.
15 C.D. Naylor, *Private Practice, Public Payment: Canadian Medicine and the Politics of Health Insurance, 1911–1966* (Montreal: McGill-Queen's University Press, 1986).
16 Simone Sandier, "Health Service Utilization and Physician Income Trends," *Health Care Financing Review* (annual supplement) 11 (1989), 33–48.
17 Weinkauf and Linton, "Physician Payment in Canada."
18 Victor R. Fuchs and James S. Hahn, "How Does Canada Do It? A Comparison of Expenditures for Physicians' Services in the United States and Canada," *NEJM*, 323 (1990), 885–90.
19 Canadian Medical Association, *Taking the Pulse: The CMA Physician Resource Survey* (Ottawa: Canadian Medical Association, 1996).
20 Ontario Ministry of Health, *Submission to the Task Force*.
21 Bernard Blishen, *Doctors in Canada: The Changing World of Medical Practice* (Toronto: University of Toronto Press in association with Statistics Canada, 1991).
22 Morris Barer, Robert Evans, and Roberta Labelle, "Fee Controls as Cost Control: Tales from the Frozen North," *Milbank Quarterly*, 66 (1988), 1–64.
23 Robert Bothwell and John English, "Pragmatic Physicians: Canadian Medicine and Health Care Insurance, 1910–1945," in S.E.D. Shortt, ed., *Medicine in Canadian Society, Historical Perspectives*, 2nd ed. (Montreal: McGill-Queen's University Press, 1992), 479–93.
24 S.E.D. Shortt, "'Before the Age of Miracles': The Rise, Fall and Rebirth of General Practice in Canada, 1890–1940," in Charles Roland, ed., *Health, Disease and Medicine, Essays in Canadian History* (Toronto: Hannah Institute for the History of Medicine, 1984), 123–52.
25 Kenneth F. Clute, *The General Practitioner: A Study of Medical Education and Practice in Ontario and Nova Scotia* (Toronto: University of Toronto Press, 1963).
26 Evans, "Health Care in Canada".
27 Anne Crichton, "The Shift from Entrepreneurial to Political Power in the Canadian Health System," *Social Science and Medicine*, 10 (1976), 59–66.
28 Catherine A. Charles, "The Medical Profession and Health Insur-

ance: An Ontario Case Study," *Social Science and Medicine*, 10 (1976), 33–38.

29 Naylor, *Private Practice, Public Payment*.

30 S. Heiber and R. Deber, "Banning Extra-billing in Canada: Just What the Doctor Didn't Order," *Canadian Public Policy*, 13 (1987), 62–74.

31 Carolyn J. Tuohy, "Medical Politics after Medicare: The Ontario Case," *Canadian Public Policy*, 2 (1976), 192–209.

32 Malcolm G. Taylor, "The Canadian Health-Care System: After Medicare," in David Coburn et al., ed., *Health and Canadian Society, Sociological Perspectives*, 2nd ed. (Toronto: Fitzhenry and Whiteside, 1987), 73–101.

33 Heiber and Deber, "Banning Extra-billing in Canada."

34 Stevenson, Williams, and Vayda,"Medical Politics and Canadian Medicare."

35 H. Michael Stevenson and A. Paul Williams, "Physicians and Medicare: Professional Ideology and Canadian Health Care Policy," *Canadian Public Policy*, 11 (1985), 504–21.

36 Paul Rhodes, "Government Grants Additional Threshold Exemptions," *Ontario Medical Review*, 59 (1992), 13–14.

37 Jonathan Lomas et al., "Paying Physicians in Canada: Minding Our Ps and Qs," *Health Affairs*, 8 (1989), 80–102.

38 "Utilization Percentage Recovery Finalized," *Ontario Medical Review*, 59 (1992), 5.

39 Morris Barer, Claudia Sanmartin, and Jonathan Lomas, "Physician Expenditure Control in Canada: Reminding Our Ps and Qs." McMaster University, Centre for Health Economics and Policy Analysis. Working Paper 95–11, Hamilton, 1995.

40 Jeremiah Hurley and R. Card, "Global Physician Budgets as Common-property Resources: Some Implications for Physicians and Medical Associations," *CMAJ*, 154 (1996), 1161–8.

41 Naylor, *Private Practice, Public Payment*; Blishen, *Doctors in Canada*.

42 Stevenson, Williams, and Vayda, "Medical Politics and Canadian Medicare"; Stevenson and Williams, "Physicians and Medicare."

43 J.Murray, "Physician Satisfaction with Capitation Patients in an Academic Family Medicine Centre," *Journal of Family Practice*, 27 (1988), 108–13.

44 Raynald Pineault, A-P. Contandriopoulos, and M-A. Fournier, "Physicians' Acceptance of an Alternative to Fee-for-Service Payment: A Possible Source of Change in Quebec Medicine," *International Journal of Health Services*, 15 (1985), 419–29.

45 Jon R. Gabel and Michael A. Redisch, "Alternative Physician Payment Methods: Incentives, Efficiency, and National Health Insurance," *Milbank Memorial Fund Quarterly*, 57 (1979), 38–59.

46 Gerald B.Hickson, William A. Altemeier, and James M. Perrin, "Physician Reimbursement by Salary or Fee-for-Service: Effect on Physician Practice Behaviour in a Randomized Prospective Study," *Paediatrics*, 80 (1987), 344–50.

47 Eugene Vayda, William Mindell, and Ira M. Rutkow, "A Decade of Surgery in Canada, England and Wales, and the United States," *Archives of Surgery*, 117 (1982), 846–53; Klim McPherson et al., "Regional Variations in the Use of Common Surgical Procedures: Within and between England and Wales, Canada, and the United States of America," *Social Science and Medicine*, 15A (1981), 273–88.

48 C.R. Gaus, B.S. Cooper and C.G. Hirschman, "Contrasts in HSO and Fee-for-Service Performance," *Social Security Bulletin*, 39 (1986), 3–14.

49 John E.Ware et al., "Comparison of Health Outcomes at a Health Maintenance Organization with Those of Fee-for-Service Care, *Lancet*, 3 May 1986, 1017–22.

50 H.S. Luft, "Assessing the Evidence of HMO Performance," *Milbank Memorial Fund Quarterly*, (1980), 501–36.

51 Kathleen Ellsbury, Daniel Montano, and John Parker "Preventive Services in a Hybrid Capitation and Fee-for-Service Setting," *Journal of Family Practice*, 28 (1989), 540–4; Renaldo Battista, J.Ivan Williams and Leslie MacFarlane, "Determinants of Preventive Practices in Fee-for-Service Primary Care," *American Journal of Preventive Medicine*, 6 (1990), 6–11.

52 Brian Hutchison, Stephen Birch, and J. Gillett, "Health Service Organizations: The Evolution of Capitation-funded Physician Care in Ontario," McMaster University, Centre for Health Economics and Policy Analysis, Working Paper 96–11, Hamilton, 1996.

53 A.C. Marcus, "Mode of Payment and Identification with a Regular Doctor: A Prospective Look at Reported Use of Services," *Medical Care*, 22 (1984), 647–57.

54 M. Poland, "The Effect of Continuity of Care on the Missed Appointment Rates in a Prenatal Clinic," *Journal of Obstetric, Gynecologic, and Neonatal Nursing*, 5 (1976), 45–7; M.Becker et al., "Predicting Compliance with Paediatric Medical Regimes," *Journal of Pediatrics*, 81 (1982), 843–54.

55 R. Holloway, C.C. Matson, and D.K. Zismar, "Patient Satisfaction and

Selected Physician Behaviour: Does Type of Practice Make a Difference?" *Journal of the American Board of Family Practice,* 29 (1989), 87–92; J.P. Murray, "A Comparison of Patient Satisfaction among Prepaid and Fee-for-Service Patients," *Journal of Family Practice,* 24 (1987), 203–7.

56 Greg Stoddart and Morris Barer, "Towards Integrated Medical Resource Policies for Canada: 6. Remuneration of Physicians and Global Expenditure Policy," *CMAJ,* 147 (1992), 36.

57 Thomas Rice, "The Impact of Changing Medicare Reimbursement Rates on Physician-induced Demand," *Medical Care,* 21 (1983), 803–15.

58 Jon R. Gabel and Thomas Rice, "Reducing Public Expenditures for Physician Services: The Price of Paying Less," *Journal of Health Politics, Policy and Law,* 9 (1985), 595–609.

59 John Rizzo and David Blumenthal, "Physician Income Targets: New Evidence on an Old Controversy," *Inquiry,* 31 (1995), 394–404.

60 Barer, Evans, and Labelle, "Fee Controls as Cost Controls."

61 Gail Wilensky and Louis Rossiter, "The Relative Importance of Physician-induced Demand in the Demand for Medical Care," *Milbank Memorial Fund Quarterly,* 61 (1983), 252–77.

62 Government of Ontario, Ministry of Health, and Ontario Medical Association, *Task Force on the Use and Provision of Medical Services: Quality Assurance and Resource Management – the Medical Services Challenges for the 1990s, Final Report, Jan., 1992* (Toronto, 1992).

63 Robert Evans, "Supplier-Induced Demand: Some Empirical Evidence and Implications," in M. Perlman, ed., *The Economics of Health and Medical Care* (London: Macmillan, 1974), 162–73.

64 Robert Evans, "Finding the Levers, Finding the Courage: Lessons from Cost Containment in North America," *Journal of Health Politics, Policy and Law,* 11 (1986), 585–615; Robert Evans et al., "Controlling Health Expenditures – the Canadian Reality," *NEJM,* 320 (1989), 571–7.

65 John S. Hughes, "How Well Has Canada Contained the Costs of Doctoring?" *Journal of the American Medical Association,* 265 (1991), 2347–51.

66 André-Pierre Contandriopoulos, "Cost Containment through Payment Mechanism: The Quebec Experience," *Journal of Public Health Policy,* 7 (1986), 224–38.

67 Morris Barer and Gregory Stoddart, *Towards Integrated Medical*

Resource Policies for Canada, Report Prepared for the Federal/Provincial/Territorial Conference of Deputy Ministers of Health. June. 1991 (Ottawa, 1991).

68 Paul Wilson, Duncan Chappell, and Robyn Lincoln, "Policing Physician Abuse in B.C.: An Analysis of Current Policies," *Canadian Public Policy*, 12 (1986), 236–44.

69 Carolyn Tuohy, "Does a Claims Monitoring System Influence High-Volume Medical Practitioners? Attitudinal Data from Ontario," *Inquiry*, 19 (1982), 18–33.

70 L. Mooney, "Changes to the MRC Process: The Expedited Review," *Ontario College of Physicians and Surgeons Members Dialogue* (Sept.–Oct. 1996), 26–32.

71 Darrel Weinkauf and Gerald Rowland, "Patient Conditions at the Primary-Care Level: A Commentary on Resource Allocation," *Ontario Medical Review*, 59 (1992), 11–15, 61.

72 Charles J. Wright, "The Fee-for-Service System Should Be Replaced," *CMAJ*, 144 (1991), 901.

73 William C. Hsiao et al., "Results and Policy Implications of the Resource-based Relative Value Study," *NEJM*, 319 (1988), 881–8.

74 Jim G. Tsitandis, "Resource-Based Relative Value Schedules: Past and Present," *Ontario Medical Review*, 59 (1992), 11–16.

75 Alex Borgiel et al., "Quality of Care in Family Practice: Does Residency Training Make a Difference?" *CMAJ*, 140 (1989), 1035–43.

76 Christel Woodward et al., "Correlates of Certification in Family Medicine in the Billing Patterns of Ontario General Practitioners," *CMAJ*, 141 (1989), 897–904.

77 Morris Barer, Robert Evans, and Gregory Stoddart, "Controlling Health Care Costs by Direct Charges to Patients: Snare or Delusion?" Ontario Economic Council Occasional Paper 10, Toronto, 1979.

78 C.E. Reeder and Arthur A. Nelson, "The Differential Impact of Co-payment on Drug Use in a Medicaid Population," *Inquiry*, 22,(1985), 396–403; Stephen Soumerai et al., "Payment Restrictions for Prescription Drugs under Medicaid, Effects on Therapy, Cost, and Equity," *NEJM*, 317 (1987), 550–6.

79 G.R. Weller and Pran Manga, "The Push for Reprivatization of Health Care Services in Canada, Britain, and the United States," *Journal of Health Politics, Policy and Law*, 8 (1983), 495–518.

80 Government of Ontario, Ministry of Health, Southwestern Ontario Comprehensive Health System Planning Commission, Final Report: *Working Together to Achieve Better Health for All*. Dec. 1991.

81 Marianne Lamb et al., *Managed Care in Canada: The Toronto Hospital's Proposed Comprehensive Health Organization* (Ottawa: Canadian Hospital Association Press, 1991).

82 Karen Harvey, "Institute for Clinical Evaluative Sciences," *Ontario Medical Review*, 59 (1992), 35–6.

83 Canadian Medical Association, *Core and Comprehensive Health Care Services; A Framework for Decision-Making* (Ottawa: Canadian Medical Association, 1994).

84 Ralph Crawshaw et al., "Developing Principles for Prudent Health Care Allocation: The Continuing Oregon Experiment," *Western Journal of Medicine*, 152 (1990), 441–6.

85 College of Family Physicians of Canada, *Position Paper on Alternative Payment Mechanisms* (Toronto, 1992).

86 Jacqueline Muldoon, "Publicly Financed Competition in Health Care: Legislative Issues," *Healthcare Management Forum* (summer 1991), 39–46; Jacqueline Muldoon and Gregory Stoddart, "Publicly Financed Competition in Health Care Delivery: A Canadian Simulation Model," *Journal of Health Economics*, 8 (1989), 313–38.

87 Wendy Graham, "Primary Care Reform: A Strategy for Stability," *Ontario Medical Review*, 63 (1996), 21–7.

CHAPTER THREE

1 Dan McCaughey, "Professional Militancy: The Medical Defence Association vs. The College of Physicians and Surgeons of Ontario, 1891–1902," in Charles Roland, ed., *Health, Disease and Medicine: Essays in Canadian History* (Toronto: Hannah Institute for the History of Medicine, 1984), 98.

2 Robert Evans, "Does Canada Have Too Many Doctors? Why Nobody Loves an Immigrant Physician," *Canadian Public Policy*, 2 (1976), 148.

3 Douglas E. Angus et al., *Sustainable Health Care for Canada* (Ottawa: Queen's University of Ottawa Economic Projects, 1995).

4 Eva Ryten, "Physician-Workforce and Educational Planning in Canada: Has the Pendulum Swung Too Far?" *Canadian Medical Association Journal (CMAJ)*, 152 (1995), 1395–8.

5 Marc Baltzan, "An Unregulated Physician Supply Stabilizes Practice Size," *Annals of the Royal College of Physicians and Surgeons of Canada*, 29 (1996), 342–6.

6 David A. Kindig and Charles M. Taylor, "Growth in the International

Physician Supply 1950 through 1979," *Journal of the American Medical Association (JAMA)*, 253 (1985), 3129–32.

7 Patrick Sullivan, "Are There Too Many Doctors? CMA Seeks 'Rational' Approach to Issue," *CMAJ*, 141 (1989), 432–3.

8 Morris Barer and Gregory Stoddart, "Towards Integrated Medical Resource Policies for Canada: 7. Undergraduate Medical Training," *CMAJ*, 147 (1992), 305–12.

9 William B. Spaulding and Walter O. Spitzer, "Implications of Medical Manpower Trends in Ontario 1961–1971," Ontario Medical Review 38 (1972), 527–33.

10 Jonathan Lomas and Morris Barer, "And Who Shall Represent the Public Interest? The Legacy of Canadian Health Manpower Policy," in Robert Evans and Gregory Stoddart, eds., *Medicare at Maturity, Achievements, Lessons and Challenges* (Calgary: University of Calgary Press, 1986), 221–86.

11 Canada, Health and Welfare Canada, *Physician Manpower in Canada 1980–2000. Report of the Federal–Provincial Advisory Committee on Health Manpower* (Ottawa: Health and Welfare Canada, 1984).

12 John K. Iglehart, "The Future Supply of Physicians," *New England Journal of Medicine (NEJM)*, 314 (1986), 860–4.

13 Morris Barer and Gregory Stoddart, "Towards Integrated Medical Resource Policies for Canada: A Background Document." McMaster University, Centre for Health Economics and Policy Analysis, Working Paper 91–7, Hamilton, 1991.

14 Canadian Medical Association, *Let's Get It Right: The CMA's Action Plan, Response to the Barer/Stoddard Report* (Ottawa: Canadian Medical Association, 1992).

15 Ontario, Ministry of Health, *Ministry of Health Expenditure Control Plan, Physicians Services* (Toronto, 1993).

16 Jonathan Lomas, Gregory Stoddart, and Morris Barer, "Supply Projections as Planning: a Critical Review of Forecasting Net Physician Requirements in Canada," *Social Science and Medicine*, 20 (1985), 411–24.

17 Bernard Bloom and Osler Peterson, "Physician Manpower Expansionism: A Policy Review," *Annals of Internal Medicine*, 90 (1979), 249–56.

18 Lomas and Barer, "And Who Shall Represent the Public Interest?"

19 Orvill Adams, "Canada's Doctors: Who They Are and What They Do: Lessons from the CMA's 1986 Manpower Survey," *CMAJ*, 40 (1989), 212–21.

20 Charlotte Gray, "Managing the Supply of MDs: Opinion Divided on Ministers' Proposal to Develop a National Plan," *CMAJ*, 151 (1994), 1476–8.

21 National Ad Hoc Working Group on Physician Resource Planning, *Report of the National Ad Hoc Working Group on Physician Resource Planning* (Ottawa: Canadian Medical Association, 1995).

22 Malcolm Anderson and Mark Rosenberg, "Ontario's Underserviced Area Program Revisited: An Indirect Analysis," *Social Science and Medicine*, 30 (1990), 35–44.

23 James Rourke, "Politics of Rural Health Care: Recruitment and Retention of Physicians," *CMAJ*, 148 (1993), 1281–4.

24 Robin Carter, "The Relation between Personal Characteristics of Physicians and Practice Location in Manitoba," *CMAJ*, 136 (1987), 366–8.

25 Malcolm Brown, "Do Physicians Locate as Spatial Competition Models Predict? Evidence from Alberta," *CMAJ*, 148 (1993), 1301–7.

26 Mary Fruen and James Cantwell, "Geographic Distribution of Physicians: Past Trends and Future Influences," *Inquiry*, 19 (1982), 44–50.

27 D.P. Forster, "The Relationships between Health Needs, Socio-environmental Indices, General Practitioner Resources and Utilization," *Journal of Chronic Diseases*, 32 (1979), 333–7.

28 Stephen Birch and Alan Maynard, "Regional Distribution of Family Practitioner Services: Implications for National Health Service Equity and Efficiency," *Journal of the Royal College of General Practice*, 37 (1987), 537–9.

29 Morris Barer and Gregory Stoddart, "Towards Integrated Medical Resource Policies for Canada: 8. Geographic Distribution of Physicians," *CMAJ*, 147 (1982), 617–23.

30. Noralou Roos, Michael Gaumont, and John Horne, "The Impact of the Physician Surplus on the Distribution of Physicians across Canada," *Canadian Public Policy*, 2 (1976), 169–91.

31 Lomas, Stoddart, and Barer, "Supply Projections as Planning."

32 William J. Copeman, "The Underserviced Area Program of the Ministry of Health of Ontario," *Canadian Family Physician*, 33 (1987), 1683–5.

33 Anderson and Rosenberg, "Ontario's Underserviced Area Program Revisited."

34 Jonathan Lomas and Gregory Stoddart, "Estimates of the Potential Impact of Nurse Practitioners on Future Requirements for Physicians

in Office-Based General Practice, *Canadian Journal of Public Health*, 76 (1985), 119–23.

35 Morris Barer, "Regulating Physician Supply: The Evolution of British Columbia's Bill 41," *Journal of Health Politics, Policy and Law*, 13 (1988), 2–25.

36 Jeremiah Hurley, "Simulated Effects of Income-Based Policies on the Distribution of Physicians," *Med Care*, 28 (1990), 221–38.

37 Barer and Stoddart, "Towards Integrated Medical Resource Policies for Canada."

38 Canadian Medical Association, *Let's Get It Right.*

39 Ontario, Ministry of Health, Report of the Steering Committee, Public Hospitals Act Review, *Into the 21st Century, Ontario Public Hospitals* (Toronto, 1992)

40 Carter, "The Relation between Personal Characteristics of Physicians and Practice Location."

41 Patrick Sullivan, "New, Validated Totals of MDs in Each Speciality Invaluable, CMA Says," *CMAJ*, 142 (1990), 1419–20.

42 Stephen Birch and John Eyles, "Needs-Based Planning of Health Care: A Critical Appraisal of the Literature," McMaster University, Centre for Health Economics and Policy Analysis, Working Paper 91–5, Hamilton, 1991.

43 Lomas and Barer, "And Who Shall Represent the Public Interest?"

44 Birch and Eyles, "Needs-Based Planning of Health Care."

45 Ontario, Premier's Council on Health Strategy, *Local Decision Making for Health and Social Services, Report on the Integration and Co-ordination Committee* (Toronto: 1992).

46 Ontario, Ministry of Health Southwestern Ontario Comprehensive Health System Planning Commission, *Working Together to Achieve Better Health for All*, Final report. (Toronto, 1991), 175.

47 Marianne Lamb et al., *Managed Care in Canada, The Toronto Hospital's Proposed Comprehensive Health Organization* (Ottawa: Canadian Hospital Association Press, 1991).

48 H. Michael Stevenson and R. Paul Williams, "Physicians and Medicare: Professional Ideology and Canadian Health Care Policy," *Canadian Public Policy*, 11 (1985), 504–21; Raynald Pinault, A.-P. Contandriopoulos, and M.-A.Fourier, "Physicians' Acceptance of an Alternative to Fee-for-Service: A Possible Source of Change in Quebec Medicine," *International Journal of Health Services*, 15 (1985), 419–29.

49 A.-P.Contandriopoulos and M.-A. Fournier, "Towards an Integrated

Medical Human Resources Management Policy for Canada: The Situation in Quebec," Appendix B; Barer and Stoddart, "Towards Integrated Medical Resource Policies for Canada."

CHAPTER FOUR

1 T.A. Brennan et al.,"Incidence of Adverse Events and Negligence in Hospitalized Patients," *New England Journal of Medicine* (*NEJM*), 324 (1991), 370–6.
2 Eugene Vayda, William Mindell, and Ira Rutkow, "A Decade of Surgery in Canada, England and Wales, and the United States," *Archives of Surgery*, 117 (1982), 846–53.
3 Eugene Vayda et al.,"Five-Year Study of Surgical Rates in Ontario's Counties," *Canadian Medical Association Journal* (*CMAJ*), 131 (1984), 111–15.
4 Steven Schroeder, Alan Schliftman, and Thomas Piemme, "Variation among Physicians in the Use of Laboratory Tests: Relation to Quality of Care," *Medical Care*, 12 (1974), 709–13.
5 Marcia Daniels and Steven Schroeder, "Variation among Physicians in Use of Laboratory Tests II. Relations to Clinical Productivity and Outcomes of Care," *Medical Care*, 15 (1977), 482–7.
6 E. Chen and C.D. Naylor, "Variation in Hospital Length of Stay for Acute Myocardial Infarction in Ontario, Canada," *Medical Care*, 32 (1994), 420–35.
7 Carolyn Tuohy, "Does a Claims Monitoring System Influence High Volume Medical Practitioners? Attitudinal Date from Ontario," *Inquiry*, 19 (1992), 18–33.
8 Tracey Tremayne-Lloyd and Lori Stolz, "OHIP Audits: Preventive Medicine," *Ontario Medical Review*, 58 (1991), 39–41.
9 Mary Lou Harrigan, *Quality of Care: Issues and Challenges in the 90s, A Literature Review* (Ottawa: Canadian Medical Association, 1992).
10 Adam Linton and David Peachy, "Guidelines for Medical Practice: 1. The Reasons Why," *CMAJ*, 143 (1990), 485–90.
11 C.D. Naylor and P.W. Armstrong, "Guidelines for the Use of Intravenous Thrombolytic Agents in Acute Myocardial Infarction,"*CMAJ*, 140 (1989), 1289–99.
12 Antoni Basinski et al., *Detection and Management of Asymptomatic Hypercholesterolemia. A Policy Document by the Toronto Working Group on Cholesterol* (Toronto: Ontario Ministry of Health, 1989).
13 Ronald G. McAuley et al., "Five-Year Results of the Peer Assessment

Program of the College of Physicians and Surgeons of Ontario,"
CMAJ, 143 (1990), 1193–9.

14 David A. Davis et al., "Attempting to Ensure Physician Competence,"
Journal of the American Medical Association (JAMA), 263 (1990):
2041–2.

15 T. Kaigas, "Monitoring and Enhancement of Physician Performance
(MEPP): A National Initiative. Part III," *College of Physicians and Surgeons of Ontario Members' Dialogue* (Sept.–Oct. 1996), 21-4.

16 Kathleen Lohr, Karl Yordy, and Samuel Thier, "Current Issues in
Quality of Care," *Health Affairs*, 7 (1988), 5–18.

17 R. Heather Palmer, "The Challenge and Prospects for Quality Assessment and Assurance in Ambulatory Care," *Inquiry*, 25 (1988),
119–31.

18 Donald Berwick, "Health Services Research and Quality of Care:
Assignment for the 1990's," Med Care 27(1989):763–771.

19 David Eddy and John Billings, "The Quality of Medical Evidence:
Implications for Quality of Care," *Health Affairs*, 7 (1988), 19–32.

20 Donald Berwick and Marion Knapp, "Theory and Practice for Measuring Health Care Quality," *Health Care Financing Review*, supplement (1987), 49–55.

21 Martin J. Bass et al., "The Physician's Actions and the Outcome of Illness in Family Practice," *Journal of Family Practice*, 23 (1986), 46, 47.

22 Alex E. Borgeil et al., "Assessing the Quality of Care in Family Physicians' Practices," *Canadian Family Physician*, 3 (1985), 853–62.

23 P.D. Cleary and B.J. McNeil, "Patient Satisfaction as an Indicator of
Quality Care," *Inquiry*, 25 (1988), 25–36.

24 Avedis Donabedian, "Twenty Years of Research on the Quality of
Medical Care, 1964–1984," *Evaluation and the Health Professions*, 8
(1985), 243–65.

25 B.A. Hulka et al., "Peer Review in Ambulatory Care: Use of Explicit
Criteria and Implicit Judgements," *Medical Care*, 17, supplement
(1979), 1–73.

26 R. Heather Palmer,"Quality Management in Ambulatory Care," in
J.B. Couch, ed., *Health Care Quality Management for the 21st Century*
(Tampa, Fla.: American College of Physician Executives, American
College of Medical Quality, 1991), 75–103.

27 Stephen Rosenberg et al., "An Eclectic Approach to Quality Control
in Fee-for-Service Health Care: The New York City Medicaid Experiment," *American Journal of Public Health*, 66 (1976), 21–30.

28 John Kelly and James Swartwout, "Development of Practice Parame-

ters by Physician Organizations," *Quality Review Bulletin*, 16 (1990), 54–7.

29 Charles Osborne and Hugh Thompson, "Criteria for Evaluation of Ambulatory Child Health Care by Chart Audit: Development and Testing of a Methodology," *Pediatrics*, 56, supplement (1976), 625–92.

30 Sheldon Greenfield et al., "Peer Review by Criteria Mapping: Criteria for Diabetes Mellitus, the Use of Decision Making in Chart Audit," *Annals of Internal Medicine*, 8 (1975), 761–70.

31 Sheldon Greenfield et al., "Comparison of a Criteria Map to a Criteria List in Quality-of-care Assessment for Patients with Chest Pain: The Relation of Each to Outcome," *Medical Care*, 19 (1981), 255–72.

32 Alvin Mushlin and Francis Appel, "Testing an Outcome-Based Quality Assurance Strategy in Primary Care," *Medical Care*, 18, supplement (1980), 1–100.

33 Barbara Woo et al., "Screening Procedures in the Asymptomatic Adult, Comparison of Physicians' Recommendations, Patients' Desires, Published Guidelines, and Actual Practice," *JAMA*, 254 (1985), 1480–4.

34 Jonathan Lomas et al., "Do Practice Guidelines Guide Practice? The Effect of a Consensus Statement on the Practice of Physicians," *NEJM*, 321 (1989), 1306–11.

35 Mark Eckman, John Wong, and Stephen Pauker, "The Role of a Clinical Decision Analysis in Medical Quality Management," in J.B.Couch, ed., *Health Care Quality Management for the 21st Century* (Tampa, Fla.: American College of Physician Executives, American College of Medical Quality, 1991), 253–80.

36 John Ware et al., "Defining and Measuring Patient Satisfaction with Medical Care," *Evaluation and Program Planning*, 6 (1983), 247–63.

37 A.R. Tarlov et al. "The Medical Outcomes Study: An Application of Methods for Monitoring the Results of Medical Care," *JAMA*, 262 (1989), 925–30.

38 Steven Woolf, "Practice Guidelines: A New Reality in Medicare. I. Recent Developments," *Archives of Internal Medicine*, 150 (1990), 1811–18.

39 John Kelly, "Practice Parameter Development by Physician Organizations," in J.B.Couch, ed., *Health Care Quality Management for the 21st Century* (Tampa, Fla.: American College of Physician Executives and American College of Medical Quality, 1991), 398–414.

40 Robert Brook, "Practice Guidelines and Practicing Medicine: Are They Compatible?" *JAMA*, 262 (1989), 3027–30.

41 Jacqueline Kosecoff et al., "Effects of the National Institutes of Health Consensus Development Program on Physician Practice," *JAMA*, 258 (1987), 2708–13.

42 Jonathan Lomas et al., "The Role of Evidence in the Consensus Process, Results from a Canadian Consensus Exercise," *JAMA*, 259 (1988), 3001–5.

43 David Eddy, "Clinical Policies and the Quality of Clinical Practice," *NEJM*, 307 (1982), 343–7.

44 Elliott Antman et al., "A Comparison of Results of Meta-analyses of Randomized Control Trials and Recommendations of Clinical Experts, Treatment for Myocardial Infarction," *JAMA*, 268 (1992), 240–8.

45 Anne-Marie Audet, Sheldon Greenfield, and Marilyn Field, "Medical Practice Guidelines: Current Activities and Future Directions," *Annals of Internal Medicine*, 113 (1990), 709–14.

46 B. Ferrier et al., "Clinical Practice Guidelines: New-to-practice Family Physicians Attitudes," *Canadian Family Physician*, 42 (1996):463–467.

47 Roberto Grilli et al., "Physicians' View of Practice Guidelines. A Survey of Italian Physicians," *Social Science and Medicine*, 43 (1996), 1283–7.

48 Joel Schectman et al., "The Effect of an Education and Feedback Intervention Group-model and Network Model Health Maintenance Organization Physician Prescribing Behavior," *Medical Care*, 33 (1995),139–44.

49 D.R. Montoya, "Impact of Feedback on Ankle X-ray Utilization Patterns in a Group of Full-time Emergency Physicians," *Annals of the Royal College of Physicians and Surgeons of Canada*, 29 (1996), 407–10.

50 Jerry Avorn, "Improving Drug-Therapy Decisions through Educational Outreach: A Randomized Controlled Trial of Academically Based 'Detailing,'" *NEJM*, 308 (1983), 1457–63; Jerry Avorn and Stephen Soumerai, "Use of Computer-Based Medicaid Drug Data to Analyze and Correct Inappropriate Medication Use," *Journal of Medical Systems*, 6 (1982), 377–86.

51 William Schaffner et al., "Improving Antibiotic Prescribing in Office Practice: A Controlled Trial of Three Educational Methods," *JAMA*, 250 (1983),1728–32; Wayne Ray et al., "Improving Antibiotic Prescribing in Outpatient Practice: Nonassociation of Outcome with

Prescriber Characteristics and Measures of Receptivity," *Medical Care,* 23 (1985),1307–13.

52 Kathleen Lohr, Robert Brook, and Michael Kaufman, "Quality of Care in the New Mexico Medicaid Program (1971–1975): The Effect of the New Mexico Experimental Medical Care Review Organization on the Use of Antibiotics for Common Infectious Diseases," *Medical Care* 18, supplement (1980).

53 William Tierney, Michael Miller, and Clement Mcdonald, "The Effect on Test Ordering of Informing Physicians of the Charges for Outpatient Diagnostic Tests," *NEJM,* 322 (1990),1499–504; Mark Chassin and Sally McCue, "A Randomized Trial of Medical Quality Assurance: Improving Physicians' Use of Pelvimetry," *JAMA,* 256 (1986), 1012–16; Steven Schroeder et al., "Use of Laboratory Tests and Pharmaceutical: Variations among Physicians and Effect of Cost Audit on Subsequent Use," *JAMA,* 225 (1973), 969–73.

54 George Everettet al., "Effect of Cost Education, Cost Audits, and Faculty Chart Review on the Use of Laboratory Services," *Archives of Internal Medicine,* 143 (1983), 942–4; F.G.R. Fowkes et al., "Trial of Strategy for Reducing the Use of Laboratory Tests," *British Medical Journal,* 292 (1986), 883–5.

55 R. Heather Palmer et al., "A Method for Evaluating Performance of Ambulatory Pediatric Tasks," *Pediatrics,* 73 (1984), 269–77; R. Heather Palmer et al., "Quality Assurance in Eight Adult Medicine Group Practices," *Medical Care,* 22 (1984), 632–43.

56 R. Heather Palmer et al., "A Randomized Trial of Quality Assurance in Sixteen Ambulatory Care Practises," *Medical Care,* 23 (1985), 751–71; R. Heather Palmer, "Does Quality Assurance Improve Ambulatory Care? Implementing a Randomized Controlled Trial in Group Practices," *Journal of Ambulatory Care Management,* 9 (1986), 1–15.

57 G. Octo. Barnett et al., "Quality Assurance through Automated Monitoring and Concurrent Feedback Using a Computer-Based Medical Information System," *Medical Care,* 16 (1978), 962–71.

58 R.N. Winickoff et al., "Improving Physician Performance through Peer Comparison Feedback," *Medical Care,* 22 (1984), 527–34.

59 Beverly Payne et al., "Method of Evaluating and Improving Ambulatory Medical Care," *Health Services Research,* 19 (1984), 218–45.

60 Jonathan Lomas et al., "Turning Practice Guidelines into Actual Practice: A Randomized Controlled Trial of Opinion Leaders and Audit/Feedback in Community Hospitals," McMaster University Cen-

tre for Health Economics and Policy Analysis, Working Paper 90-16,
1990, Hamilton, Ont.

61 Kathleen Lohr and Steven Schroeder, "A Strategy for Quality Assur-
ance in Medicare," *NEJM*, 322 (1990), 707–12; Thomas Morford,
"Federal Efforts to Improve Peer Review Organizations," *Health
Affairs*, 8 (1989), 174–8.

62 J.E. Casanova, "Status of Quality Assurance Programs in American
Hospitals," *Medical Care*, 28 (1990), 1104–9.

63 Kathryn Harvey, "Institute for Clinical Evaluative Sciences," *Ontario
Medical Review*, 59 (1992), 35–6.

64 Adam Linton and C.D. Naylor, "Organized Medicine and the Assessment of Technology: Lessons from Ontario," *NEJM*, 323 (1990),
1463–7.

65 Ontario, Ministry of Health, Public Hospitals Act Review, *Into the
21st Century: Ontario Public Hospitals,* Report of the Steering Committee (Toronto, 1992).

66 Lucian L. Leape, "Practice Guidelines and Standards: An Overview,"
Quality Review Bulletin (1990), 45.

67 R. Baker and L. Green, "Quality Assurance for Family Practice
Trainees in the USA and the UK: Too Little Too Late?" *Medical Education*, 24 (1990), 258–63.

68 Marianne Lamb et al., *Managed Care in Canada: The Toronto Hospital's
Proposed Comprehensive Health Organization* (Ottawa: Canadian Hospital Association Press, 1991).

69 Ontario, Ministry of Health, Southwestern Ontario Comprehensive
Health System Planning Commission, *Working Together to Achieve Better
Health for All,* Final Report (Toronto, 1991).

70 Health Services Research Group, "Studying Patients' Preferences in
Health Care Decision Making," *CMAJ*, 147 (1992), 859–64.

71 Helen Winefield, Timothy Murrell, and Julie Clifford, "Process and
Outcomes in General Practice Consultations: Problems in Defining
High Quality Care," *Social Science and Medicine*, 41 (1995), 969–75.

72 M.A. Morehead, "The Medical Audit as an Operational Tool," *American Journal of Public Health*, 57 (1967), 1643.

73 Avedis Donabedian, "Quality and Cost: Choices and Responsibilities," *Inquiry*, 25 (1988), 97.

CHAPTER FIVE

1 Stephen Shortell, Michael Morrisey, and Douglas Conrad, "Economic Regulation and Hospital Behaviour: The Effects on Medical Staff

Organization and Hospital–Physician Relationships," *Health Services Research*, 20 (1985), 597–628.

2 Christopher Wilson, *New on Board: Essentials of Governance for Hospital Trustees* (Ottawa: Canadian Hospital Association Press, 1991); W. Vickery Stoughton, "DRGs from a Canadian Standpoint," *Health Care*, 25 (1983), 13–14.

3 Canada, Department of Finance, *Federal-Provincial Study on the Cost of Government and Expenditure Management* (Ottawa, 1992); Ontario, Ministry of Treasury and Economics, "Managing Health Care Resources, Meeting Ontario's Priorities," 1992 Ontario Budget Supplementary paper (Toronto, 1992).

4 V.V. Murray, T.D. Jick, and P. Bradshaw, "Hospital Funding Constraints: Strategic and Tactical Decision Responses to Sustained Moderate Levels of Crisis in Six Canadian Hospitals," *Social Science and Medicine*, 18 (1984), 211–19.

5 J.R. Lave, P. Jacobs, and F. Markel, "Transitional Funding: Changing Ontario's Global Budget System," *Health Care Financing Review*, 13 (1992), 77–84.

6 J.R. Lave, P.J. Jacobs, and F. Markel, "Ontario's Hospital Transitional Funding Initiative: An Overview and Assessment," *Health Care Management Forum*, 4 (1991), 3–21; Ontario Hospital Association, *Development of a Case Costing Methodology for Ontario Hospitals. Phase One: Feasibility and Advisability* (Toronto: Ontario Hospital Association in association with the Ontario Ministry of Health, 1991).

7 Allan Detsky, Sidney Stacey, and Claire Bombardier, "The Effectiveness of a Regulatory Strategy in Containing Hospital Costs: The Ontario Experience, 1967–1981," *New England Journal of Medicine (NEJM)*, 309 (1983), 151–9.

8 Allan Detsky et al., "Containing Ontario's Hospital Costs under Universal Insurance in the 1980's: What Was the Record?" *Canadian Medical Association Journal (CMAJ)*, 142 (1990), 565–72.

9 Geoffrey Anderson, Joseph Newhouse, and Leslie Roos, "Hospital Care for Elderly Patients with Diseases of the Circulatory System: A Comparison of Hospital Use in the United States and Canada," *NEJM*, 321 (1989), 1443–8; Jean L. Rouleau et al., "A Comparison of Management Patterns after Acute Myocardial Infarction in Canada and the United States," *NEJM*, 328 (1993), 779–84.

10 Joseph Newhouse, Geoffrey Anderson, and Leslie Roos, "Hospital Spending in the United States and Canada," *Health Affairs*, 7 (1988), 6–16; D.A. Redelmeire and V.R. Fuchs, "Hospital Expenditures in the United States and Canada," *NEJM*, 328 (1993), 772–8.

11 Ontario, Ministry of Health, *Program Review of Hospital Expenditures, Background, and Analysis* (Toronto, 1991).

12 Health Services Research Group, "Small-Area Variations: What Are They and What Do They Mean?" *CMAJ*, 146 (1992), 467–70; P. Paul-Shaheen, J.D. Clark, and D. Williams, "Small Area Analysis: A Review and Analysis of the North American Literature," *Journal of Health Politics, Policy and Law*, 12 (1987), 741– 809.

13 Steven Schroeder, Alan Schliftman, and Thomas Piemme, "Variation among Physicians in Use of Laboratory Tests: Relation to Quality of Care," *Medical Care*, 12 (1974), 709–13; Marcia Daniels and Steven Schroeder, "Variation among Physicians in Use of Laboratory Tests II: Relation to Clinical Productivity and Outcome of Care," *Medical Care*, 15 (1977), 482–7; David Hardwick et al., "Clinical Styles and Motivation: A Study of Laboratory Test Use," *Medical Care*, 13 (1975), 397–407.

14 Regis Blais, "Variations in Surgical Rates in Quebec: Does Access to Teaching Hospitals Make a Difference?" *CMAJ*, 148 (1993), 1729–36.

15 Eugene Vayda, "Four-Year Study of Surgical Rates in Ontario's Counties," *CMAJ*, 131 (1984), 111–15.

16 Mark Chassin et al., Variations in the Use of Medical and Surgical Services by the Medicare Population," *NEJM*, 314 (1986), 285–90.

17 Eugene Vayda, William Mindell, and Ira Rutkow, "A Decade of Surgery in Canada, England and Wales, and the United States," *Archives of Surgery*, 117 (1982), 846–53.

18 Mark Chassin et al., "Does Inappropriate Use Explain Geographic Variations in the Use of Health Care Services? A Study of Three Procedures," *Journal of the Americal Medical Association (JAMA)*, 258 (1987), 2533–37; Lucian Leape et al., "Does Inappropriate Use Explain Small-Area Variations in the Use of Health Care Services?" *JAMA*, 263 (1990), 669–72.

19 Klim McPherson et al., "Regional Variations in the Use of Common Surgical Procedures: Within and between England and Wales, Canada and the United States of America," *Social Science and Medicine*, 15A (1981), 273–88.

20 Daniel Cherkin et al., "The Use of Medical Resources by Residency–Trained Family Physicians and General Internists: Is There a Difference?" *Medical Care*, 25 (1987), 455–69.

21 J.M. Eisenberg, "Physician Utilization: The State of Research about Physicians' Practice Patterns," *Medical Care*, 25 (1985), 461–83.

22 John E.F. Hastings et al., "An Interim Report on the Sault Ste. Marie Study: A Comparison of Personal Health Services Utilization," *Canadian Journal of Pubic Health*, 61 (1970), 289–96.

23 Noralou Roos et al., "Variations in Physicians' Hospitalization Practices: A Population-Based Study in Manitoba, Canada," *American Journal of Public Health*, 76 (1986), 45–51.

24 G. Ross Langley et al., "Effects of Nonmedical Factors on Family Physicians' Decisions about Referral for Consultation," *CMAJ*, 147 (1992), 659–66.

25 Darrel Weinkauf and Gerald Rowland, "Who Initiates Contact with the Primary-Care Practitioner? An Ontario Survey of Physicians' Perceptions," *Ontario Medical Review*, 58 (1991), 24–31.

26 Morris Barer et al., "Aging and Health Care Utilization: New Evidence on Old Fallacies," *Social Science and Medicine*, 24 (1987), 851–62.

27 Pran Manga, Robert Brogles, and Douglas Angus, "The Determinants of Hospital Utilization under a Universal Public Insurance Program in Canada," *Medical Care*, 25 (1987), 658–70; Robert Brogles et al., "The Use of Physician Services under a National Health Insurance Scheme: An Examination of the Canada Health Survey," *Medical Care*, 21 (1983), 1037–54.

28 Stanley Shapiro et al., "Long-term Adult Use of Ambulatory Services Provided by Physicians in a Canadian Medical Care Plan," *Medical Care*, 24 (1986), 418–28.

29 Charlotte Muller, "Review of Twenty Years Research on Medical Care Utilization," *Health Services Research*, 21 (1986), 129–44.

30 Ron Giegle and Stanley Jones, "Outcomes Measurement: A Report from the Front," *Inquiry*, 27 (1990), 7–13; Health Services Research Group, "Outcomes and the Management of Health Care," *CMAJ*, 147 (1992), 1775–80.

31 Kathleen Lohr, "Outcome Measurement: Concepts and Questions," *Inquiry*, 25 (1988), 37–47.

32 A.R. Tarlov et al., "The Medical Outcome Study: An Application of Methods for Monitoring the Results of Medical Care," *JAMA*, 262 (1989), 925–30; S. Greenfield, "The Use of Outcomes in Medical Practice Applications of the Medical Outcomes Study," in J.B. Couch, ed. , *Health Care Quality Management for the 21st Century* (Tampa, Fla.: American College of Physician Executives, American College of Medical Quality, 1991).

33 John Wennberg, "Outcomes Research, Cost Containment, and the Fear of Health Care Rationing," *NEJM*, 323 (1990), 1202–4.

34 Geoffrey Anderson, Sam Sheps, and K.Cardiff, "Hospital-based Utilization Management: A Cross Canada Survey," *CMAJ*, 143 (1990),
1025–30.

35 S.B. Sheps, Geoffrey Anderson, and K. Cardiff, "Utilization Management: A Literature Review for Canadian Health Care Administrators," *Health Care Management Forum*, 4 (1991), 34–9.

36 F.P. Harrison, D. Juzwishin, and R. Roger, "Quality of Care and Utilization Management: Contemporary Tools and Strategies," *Health
Care Management Forum*, 2 (1989), 18–23.

37 F.P. Harrison and W.F. Roger, "Quality Utilization Management: Preliminary Results to a Canadian Approach," *Health Care Management
Forum*, 3 (1990), 28–33.

38 Rhonda Cockerill et al., "Planning the Role of a Hospital," *Canadian
Health Care Management*, 2 (1989), 1–15.

39 Donald Carlow and Patricia Rae, "Physician Impact Analysis: An
Imperative for the Modern Hospital," *Health Care Management Forum*,
1 (1988), 22–7; Roberta Shapiro and Gerald Glandon, "Medical
Staff Planning: An Approach to Managing Critical Hospital Assets,"
Health Care Management Review, 9 (1984), 27–40.

40 Ontario Hospital Association, *Guidelines for Medical Manpower Planning and Impact Analysis in Hospitals* (Toronto, 1991).

41 Dieter Kuntz et al., "Revisiting Physician Impact Analyses: Predict-
ed versus Observed Hospital Resource Use," *Health Care Management Forum*, 6 (1993), 27–33; Jacqueline Roberts et al., "Physician
Impact Analysis Predictions in Ontario Hospitals: Does the Emper-
or Have Clothes?" *Health Care Management Forum*, 9 (1996),
35–42.

42 Ontario, Ministry of Health, Public Hospitals Act Review, *Into the 21st
Century. Ontario Public Hospitals*, Report of the Steering Committee
(Toronto, 1992).

43 Ontario, Ministry of Health, *Working Together to Achieve Better Health for
All*, Report of the Southwestern Ontario Comprehensive Health Systems Planning Commission (Toronto, 1991).

44 Marianne Lamb et al., *Managed Care in Canada: The Toronto Hospital's
Proposed Comprehensive Health Organization* (Ottawa: Canadian Hospital Association Press, 1991).

45 Ralph Sutherland and Jane Fulton, *Health Care in Canada: A Description and Analysis of Canadian Health Services* (Ottawa: The Health
Group, 1990); Cindy Orsund-Gassiot and Sharon Lindsey, *Handbook
of Medical Staff Management* (Gaithersburg, Md.: Aspen Publishers,

1990); Lawrence Wolper and J.J. Pena, *Health Care Administration* (Rockville, Md.: Aspen Publishers, 1987).

46 Enrique Ruelas and Peggy Leatt, "The Roles of Physician-Executives in Hospitals: A Framework for Management Education," *Journal of Health Administration Education*, 3 pt.2 (1985), 151–69.

47 Stuart Marylander, "Management Professionals vs. Medical Professionals," in J.O. Hepner, ed., *Hospital Administrator-Physician Relationships* (St. Louis, Mo.: C.V. Mosby, 1980), 11–17; J.A. Raelin, *The Clash of Cultures: Managers Managing Professionals* (Boston: Harvard Business School Press, 1991).

48 Paul Meyer and Stephen Tucker, "Incorporating an Understanding of Independent Practice Physician Culture into Hospital Structure and Operations," *Hospital and Health Services Administration*, 37 (1992), 465–76.

49 Sandra Gill, "Can Doctors and Administrators Work Together," *Physician Executive*, 13 (1987), 11–16.

50 R.R. Alford, *Health Care Politics: Ideological and Interest Group Barriers to Reform* (Chicago: University of Chicago Press, 1975).

51 Paul Starr, *The Social Transformation of American Medicine* (New York: Basic Books, 1982).

52 John McKinlay and John Stoeckle, "Corporatization and the Social Transformation of Doctoring," *International Journal of Health Services*, 18 (1988), 191–205.

53 Michael Wahn, "The Decline of Medical Dominance in Hospitals," in David Coburn et. al., eds., *Health and Canadian Society, Sociological Perspectives*, 2nd ed. (Toronto: Fitzhenry and Whiteside, 1987), 422–40.

54 Robert Boissoneau, Frank Williams, and Janet Cowley, "Matrix Organization Increases Physician, Management Cooperation," *Hospital Progress*, 65 (1984), 54–7.

55 Peter Ellis and Patrick Gaskin, "Sunnybrook's Matrix Organizational Model – Moving Ahead," *Health Care Management Forum*, 1 (1988), 12–15.

56 Bruce Harber and Godwin Eni, "Issues for Consideration in the Establishment of a Program Management Structure," *Health Care Management Forum*, 2 (1989), 6–13, 38.

57 Simon Capewell, "Clinical Directorates: A Panacea for Clinicians Involved in Management?" *Health Bulletin*, 50 (1992), 441–7.

58 Hospital Medical Records Institute, *Final Report: HMRI Resource Intensity Weight 1990 Re-development Project* (Toronto, 1990); Hospital Medical Records Institute, *HMRI 1991 Resource Intensity Weights, Summary*

of Methodology (Toronto, 1991); Eric Fonberg and Denis MacDonald, *A Physician's Guide to Hospital Data* (Toronto: Hospital Medical Records Institute, 1992).

59 W.M. Tierney, M.E. Miller, and C.J. McDonald, "The Effect on Test Ordering of Informing Physicians of the Charges for Outpatient Diagnostic Tests," *NEJM*, 322 (1990), 1499–1504.

60 Kant Patel, "Physicians and DRGs, Hospital Management Alternatives," *Evaluation and the Health Professions*, 11 (1988), 487–505.

61 Sandford Weiner et al., "Economic Incentives and Organizational Realities: Managing Hospitals under DRGs," *Millbank Quarterly*, 65 (1987), 463–87.

62 Charles Botz, "Weighting Case Mix Groups: The Fatal Flaw in Resource Intensity Weights," *Health Care Management Forum*, 2 (1989), 8–11.

63 Charles Botz, "Principles for Funding on a Case Mix Basis: Construction of Case Weights (RIWs)," *Health Care Management Forum*, 4 (1991), 22–32.

64 Noralou Roos and Jean Freeman, "Potential for Inpatient–Outpatient Substitution with Diagnosis-Related Groups," *Health Care Financing Review*, 10 (1989), 31–8.

65 Carol Thomas, "Physician-Managers and Budget Control," *Canadian Health Care Management*, 37 supplement (1989), 33–8.

66 Bernard Perey, "The Role of the Physician Manager," *Health Management Forum*, 5 (1984), 48–55.

67 Peter Morgan and Lynn Cohen, "Can Physicians Afford Not to Get Involved in Hospital Administration?" *CMAJ*, 146 (1992), 751–4; Michael Redisch, "Physician Involvement in Hospital Decision Making," in John B. McKinlay, ed., *Health Care Consumers, Professionals, and Organizations* (Cambridge, Mass.: MIT Press, 1981), 337–63.

68 David Kindig and Nancy Dunham, "How Much Administration Is Today's Physician Doing?" *Physician Executive*, 17 (1991), 3–7.

69 Anne Gilmore, "Taking Care of Business: MDs in Search of Management Skills Turning to MBA Courses," *CMAJ*, 146 (1992), 743–7.

70 Orvill Adams, "Getting Physicians Involved in Hospital Management," *CMAJ*, 134 (1986), 157–9.

71 Joan Eakin, "Hospital Power Structure and the Democratization of Hospital Administration in Quebec," *Social Science and Medicine*, 18 (1984), 221–8.

72 J. E. Casanova, "Status of Quality Assurance Programs in American Hospitals," *Medical Care*, 28 (1990), 1104–9.

CHAPTER SIX

1 Stanley J. Reiser, *Medicine and the Reign of Technology* (Cambridge: Cambridge University Press, 1978), x.

2 Renaldo N. Battista, "Innovation and Diffusion of Health Related Technologies: A Conceptual Framework," *International Journal of Technology Assessment in Health Care*, 5 (1989), 227–48.

3 Louise Russell, "Regulating the Diffusion of Hospital Technologies," *Law and Contemporary Problems*, 43 (1979), 26–42.

4 Konrad Kressley, "Diffusion of High Technology Medical Care and Cost Control: A Public Policy Dilemma," *Technology in Society*, 3 (1981), 305–22.

5 Peter Neuman, Soheyla Gharib, and Milton Weinstein, "The Cost of Successful Delivery with In Vitro Fertilization," *New England Journal of Medicine (NEJM)*, 331(1994), 239–43.

6 Paul Heckerling and Marion Verp, "A Cost-effectiveness Analysis of Amniocentesis and Chorionic Villus Sampling for Prenatal Genetic Testing," *Medical Care*, 32 (1994), 863–80.

7 Allan Detsky et al., "Containing Ontario's Hospital Costs under Universal Insurance in the 1980's: What Was the Record?" *Canadian Medical Association Journal (CMAJ)*, 142 (1990), 565–72.

8 D.A. Redelmeier and V.R. Fuchs, "Hospital Expenditures in the United States and Canada," *NEJM*, 328 (1993), 772–8.

9 Joseph Newhouse, Geoffrey Anderson, and Leslie Roos, "Hospital Spending in the United States and Canada: A Comparison," *Health Affairs*, 7 (1988), 6–16.

10 Allan Detsky and I.G. Naglie, "A Clinician's Guide to Cost-effectiveness Analysis," *Annals of Internal Medicine*, 113 (1990), 147–54.

11 Jonathan Showstack, Steven Schroeder, and Michael Matsumota, "The Changes in the Use of Medical Technologies, 1972–1977: A Study of Ten Inpatient Diagnoses," *NEJM*, 306 (1982), 706–12.

12 Anne Scitovsky, "Changes in the Costs of Treatment of Selected Illnesses, 1971–1981," *Medical Care*, 23(1985), 1345–56.

13 Thomas Moloney and David Rogers, "Medical Technology: A Different View of the Contentious Debate over Costs," *NEJM*, 301 (1979), 1413–19.

14 David Feeny, "New Health Care Technologies: Their Effect on Health and the Cost of Health Care," in David Feeny, Gordon Guyatt, and Peter Tugwell, eds., *Health Care Technology: Effectiveness, Effi-*

ciency and Public Policy (Montreal: Canadian Medical Association and Institute for Research on Public Policy, 1986), 5–24.

15 Stephen Shortell et al., "The Performance of Intensive Care Units: Does Good Management Make a Difference?" *Medical Care*, 32 (1994), 508–25.

16 Thomas McKeown, *The Role of Medicine: Dream, Mirage or Nemesis?* (Princeton, NJ: Princeton University Press, 1979).

17 E.C. Lambert, *Modern Medical Mistakes* (Toronto: Fitzhenry and Whiteside, 1978).

18 Louise Russell, *Educated Guesses: Making Policy about Medical Screening Tests* (Berkeley: University of California Press, 1994).

19 John McKinlay and Sonja McKinlay, "The Questionable Contribution of Medical Measures to the Decline of Mortality in the United States in the Twentieth Century," *Milbank Memorial Fund Quarterly*, 55 (1977), 405–28.

20 J.P. Bunker, H.S. Frazier, and F. Mosteller, "Improving Health: Measuring Effects of Medical Care," *Milbank Quarterly*, 72 (1994), 225–58.

21 John McKinlay, "From 'Promising Report' to `Standard Procedure': Seven Stages in the Career of a Medical Innovation," *Milbank Memorial Fund Quarterly*, 59 (1981), 374–411.

22 H. David Banta and Barbara McNeil, "Evaluation of the CAT Scanner and Other Diagnostic Technologies," *Health Care Management Review*, 1978 (winter), 7–19.

23 H. David Banta, "Embracing or Rejecting Innovations: Clinical Diffusion of Health Care Technology," in Stanley Reiser and Michael Anbar, eds., *The Machine at the Bedside, Strategies for Using Technology in Patient Care* (Cambridge: Cambridge University Press, 1984), 65–92.

24 Stephen Baker, "The Diffusion of High Technology Medical Innovation: the Computed Tomography Scanner Example," *Social Science and Medicine*, 13 (1979), 155–62.

25 Raisa Deber, Gail Thompson, and Peggy Leatt, "Technology Acquisition in Canada: Control in a Regulated Market," *International Journal of Technology Assessment in Health Care*, 4 (1988), 185–206.

26 L. Tad Cowley et al., "Magnetic Resonance Imaging Marketing and Investment: Tensions between the Forces of Business and the Practice of Medicine," *Chest*, 105 (1994), 920–8.

27 "MRI Service Expansion Unveiled," *Ontario Medical Review*, 61 (1994), 52.

28 Gary Whitted, "Medical Technology Diffusion and Its Effects on the

Modern Hospital," *Health Care Management Review*, 1981 (spring), 45–54.

29 David Feeny, "The Diffusion of New Health Care Technologies," in David Feeny, Gordon Guyatt, and Peter Tugwell, eds., *Health Care Technology: Effectiveness, Efficiency and Public Policy* (Montreal: Canadian Medical Association and Institute for Research on Public Policy, 1986), 32.

30 Robert Evans, "The Fiscal Management of Medical Technology: The Case of Canada," in H. David Banta, ed., *Resources for Health: Technology Assessment for Policy Making* (New York: Praeger, 1982), 180.

31 Raisa Deber and Gail Thompson, "Purchasing Hospital Capital Equipment: What Role for Technology Assessment?" in Raisa Deber and Gail Thompson eds., *Restructuring Canada's Health Services System: How Do We Get There from Here?* (Toronto: University of Toronto Press, 1992), 213–22.

32 Raisa Deber et al., "Technology Acquisition in Canadian Hospitals: How Is It Done, and Where Is the Information Coming From?" *Healthcare Management Forum*, 7 (1994); 18–27.

33 Anne Greer, "Rationing Medical Technology: Hospital Decision Making in the United States and England," *International Journal of Technology Assessment in Health Care*, 3 (1987), 199–222.

34 Seymour Perry, "The Brief Life of the National Center for Health Care Technology," *NEJM*, 307 (1982), 1095–1100.

35 David Blumenthal, "Federal Policy towards Health Care Technology: The Case of the National Center," *Milbank Memorial Fund Quarterly*, 61 (1983), 584–613.

36 Seymour Perry, "Technology Assessment: Continuing Uncertainty," *NEJM*, 314 (1986), 240–3.

37 Renaldo Battista, "Health Care Technology Assessment: Linking Science and Policy Making," *CMAJ*, 146 (1992), 461–2.

38 D. Menon, "Canadian Co-ordinating Office for Health Technology Assessment (CCOTHA)," in E.Clarke and D.Marshall eds., *Technology Assessment: National and International Perspectives on Research and Practice. A Satellite Symposium of the Eighth Annual Meeting of the International Society for Technology Assessment in Health Care* (Ottawa: Canadian Co-ordinating Office for Health Technology Assessment, 1992), 3–6.

39 Adam Linton and C.D. Naylor, "Organized Medicine and the Assessment of Technology: Lessons from Ontario," *NEJM*, 323 (1990), 1463–7.

40 Peter Tugwell et al., "The Measurement Iterative Loop: A Framework

for the Critical Appraisal of Need, Benefits and Costs of Health Interventions," *Journal of Chronic Diseases*, 38 (1985), 339–51; Gordon Guyattet al., "The Role of Before–After Studies of Therapeutic Impact in the Evaluation of Diagnostic Technologies," *Journal of Chronic Diseases*, 39 (1986), 295–304; Gordon Guyatt et al., "Framework for Clinical Evaluation of Diagnostic Technologies," *CMAJ*, 134 (1986), 587–94; and Gordon Guyatt et al., "Guidelines for the Clinical and Economic Evaluation of Health Care Technologies," *Social Science and Medicine*, 22 (1986), 393–408.

41   Andreas Laupacis et al., "How Attractive Does a New Technology Have to Be to Warrant Adoption and Utilization? Tentative Guidelines for Using Clinical and Economic Evaluations," *CMAJ*, 146 (1992), 473–81.

42   Amiram Gafni and Stephen Birch, "Guidelines for the Adoption of New Technologies: A Prescription for Uncontrolled Growth in Expenditures and How to Avoid the Problem," *CMAJ*, 148 (1993), 913–17.

43   C.D. Naylor et al., "Technology Assessment and Cost-Effectiveness Analysis: Misguided Guidelines?" *CMAJ*, 148 (1993), 921–4.

44. Bryan Jennett, "Assessment of Clinical Technologies: Importance for Provision and Use," *International Journal of Technology Assessment in Health Care*, 4 (1988), 435–45; Graham Loomes and Lynda McKenzie, "The Use of QALYs in Health Care Decision Making," *Social Science Medicine*, 28 (1989), 299–308; Amiram Gafni, "Measuring the Adverse Effects of Unnecessary Hypertension Drug Therapy: QALYs vs HYE," *Clinical Investigations in Medicine*, 14 (1991), 266–70; and John Hornberger, Donald Redelmeier, and Jeffrey Petersen, "Variability among Methods to Assess Patients' Well-being and Consequent Effect on a Cost-effectiveness Analysis," *Journal of Clinical Epidemiology*, 45 (1992), 505–12.

45   Neill A. Iscoe et al., "Temporal Trends in Breast Cancer Surgery in Ontario: Can One Randomized Trial Make a Difference?" *CMAJ*, 150 (1994), 1109–15.

46   M.R. Chassin and S.M. McCue, "A Randomized Trial of Medical Quality Assurance: Improving Physicians' Use of Pelvimetry," *Journal of American Medicine Association (JAMA)*, 256 (1986), 1012–16.

47   C.D. Naylor et al., "Coronary Thrombolysis – Clinical Guidelines and Public Policy: Results of an Ontario Practitioner Survey," *CMAJ*, 142 (1990), 1071–6.

48   W.W. Rosser and W.H. Palmer, "Dissemination of Guidelines on Cho-

lesterol: Effects on Patterns of Practice of General Practitioners and Family Physicians in Ontario," *Canadian Family Physician*, 39 (1993), 280–4.

49 Jonathan Lomas et al., "Do Practice Guidelines Guide Practice? The Effect of a Consensus Statement on the Practice of Physicians," *NEJM*, 321 (1989), 1306–11.

50 Jacqueline Kosecoff et al., "Effects of the National Institutes of Health Consensus Development Program on Physician Practice," *JAMA*, 258 (1987), 2708–13.

51 S.E.D. Shortt, "Physicians, Science, and Status: Issues in the Professionalization of Anglo-American Medicine in the Nineteenth Century," *Medical History*, 27 (1983), 51–68.

52 Malcolm Brown, *Health Economics and Policy, Problems and Prescriptions* (Toronto: McClelland and Stewart, 1991), 169.

53 Jane Fulton, *Canada's Health System, Bordering on the Possible* (New York: Faulkner and Gray, 1993), 139.

54 Jonathan Lomas, "Teaching Old (and Not So Old) Docs New Tricks: Effective Ways to Implement Research Findings," McMaster University Centre for Health Economics and Policy Analysis, Working Paper 93–4, Hamilton, 1993.

55 Marshall Beckner, "Factors Affecting Diffusion of Innovations among Health Professionals," *American Journal of Public Health*, 60 (1970), 294–304.

56 H.S. Luft, "Assessing the Evidence on HMO Performance," *Milbank Fund Quarterly*, 58 (1980), 501–36.

57 Stephen Birch et al., "HSO Performance: A Critical Appraisal of Current Research," McMaster University Centre for Health Economics and Policy Analysis, Working Paper 90–1, Hamilton, 1990.

58 Raisa Deber, "Translating Technology Assessment into Policy: Conceptual Issues and Tough Choices," *International Journal of Technology Assessment in Health Care*, 8 (1992), 131–7.

59 Ontario, Ministry of Health, Report of Steering Committee, Public Hospitals Act Review, *Into the 21st Century, Ontario Public Hospitals* (Toronto, 1992).

60 Anthony Romeo, Judith Wagner and Robert Lee, "Prospective Reimbursement and the Diffusion of New Technologies in Hospitals," *Journal of Health Economics*, 3 (1984), 1–24.

61 Pran Manga, "Cost-Containing Medical Technology" *Health Care Management Forum*, 2 (1989), 26–31.

62 Raisa Deber et al., "Technology Acquisition in Canadian Hospitals:

How Are We Doing?" *Healthcare Management Forum*, 8 (1995), 23–8.

63 Ontario, Ministry of Health, Southwestern Ontario Comprehensive Health System Planning Commission, *Working Together to Achieve Better Health for All*, Final Report (Toronto, 1991).

64 Michael Drummond, "Evaluation of Health Technology: Economic Issues for Health Policy and Policy Issues for Economic Appraisal," *Social Science and Medicine*, 38 (1994), 1593–1600.

65 David Feeny, "Health Technology in Ontario: Report to the Ontario Health Review Panel," McMaster University Centre for Health Economics and Policy Analysis, Working Paper 7, Hamilton, 1988.

66 H. David Banta and Louise Russell, "Policies towards Medical Technology: An International Review," *International Journal of Health Services*, 4 (1981), 631–52.

67 David Feeny and Gregory Stoddart, "Towards Improved Health Technology Policy in Canada: A Proposal for the National Health Technology Assessment Council," *Canadian Public Policy*, 14 (1988), 254–65.

68 H. David Banta and Clyde Behney, "Policy Formulation and Technology Assessment," *Milbank Memorial Fund Quarterly*, 59 (1981), 445–79; John Bunker, Jinnet Fowles, and Ralph Schaffarzick, "Evaluations of Medical-Technology Strategies, Proposal for an Institute for Health-Care Evaluation," (second of two parts), *NEJM*, 306 (1982), 687–92.

69 Harvey Fineberg, "Technology Assessment, Motivation, Capability and Future Directions," *Medical Care*, 23 (1985), 663–71.

70 Harvey Fineberg and Howard Hiatt, "Evaluation of Medical Practices: The Case for Technology Assessment," *NEJM*, 301 (1979), 1086–91.

CONCLUSION

1 R. Brennan, "Vankoughnet among MPP's to Condemn Own Party," *Kingston Whig-Standard* 28 Feb. 1997, sect 1:1, col. 5.

2 Ontario, Ministry of Health, Southwestern Ontario Comprehensive Health System Planning Commission, *Working Together to Achieve Better Health for All*, Final Report (Toronto, Dec. 1991).

3 Ted Boadway, "An Introduction to Integrated Health Systems," *Ontario Medical Review*, 64 (1997), 28–30; Ontario, Ministry of

Health, Health Services Restructuring Commission, *A Vision of Ontario's Health Sservices System* (Toronto, 1997).

4 Peggy Leatt, George Pink, and C. David Naylor, "Integrated Delivery Systems: Has Their Time Come in Canada?" *Canadian Medical Association Journal* (CMAJ), 154 (1996), 803–9.

5 Canadian Medical Association, *Taking the Pulse: The CMA Resource Survey* (Ottawa: Canadian Medical Association, 1995).

6 Jonathan Lomas, "Devolving Authority for Health in Canada's Provinces IV. Emerging Issues and Future Prospects" McMaster University, Centre for Health Economics and Policy Analysis, Working Paper 96–5, Hamilton, 1996.

7 Jonathan Lomas, G. Veenstra, and J. Woods, "Devolving Authority for Health Care in Canada's Provinces: 2. Backgrounds, Resources and Activities of Board Members," *CMAJ*, 156 (1997), 513–20.

8 Jeremiah Hurley, Stephen Birch, and John Eyles, "Geographically-Decentralized Planning and Management in Health Care: Some Informational Issues and Their Implications," *Social Science and Medicine*, 41 (1995), 3–11.

9 Raisa Deber, "International Experience with Decentralization and Regionalization, Northern Europe," in John Dorland and S. Mathwin Davis, eds., *How Many Roads? Regionalization and Decentralization in Health Care* (Kingston: Queen's University, 1996), 53–62.

10 C. David Naylor, *Private Practice, Public Payment: Canadian Medicine and the Politics of Health Insurance, 1911–1966* (Montreal: McGill-Queen's University Press, 1986).

A Note on Sources

The works consulted in the preparation of this book will be evident from the notes. However, for readers desiring a brief introduction to readily accessible journals and published monographs on Canadian, and particularily Ontario, health policy, the following material may prove useful. Publications by governments or private organizations are not included.

Three Canadian medical periodicals often provide material relevant to health policy: the *Canadian Medical Association Journal*, *Healthcare Management Forum*, and the *Ontario Medical Review*. Outside the medical field, *Canadian Public Policy* carries occasional papers on health topics. Among the most useful foreign periodicals are the following: the *International Journal of Health Services*, *Medical Care*, the (variously titled) *Milbank Quarterly*, the *New England Journal of Medicine*, and *Social Science and Medicine*.

Two research groups regularly publish working papers: McMaster University Centre for Health Economics and Policy Analysis and the Toronto-based Institute for Clinical Evaluative Sciences. A helpful summary of research from the latter is available in C. David Naylor, Geoffrey M. Anderson, and Vivek Goel, eds., *Patterns of Health Care in Ontario* (Toronto: Canadian Medical Association, 1994), and Ivek Goel, J. Ivan Williams, Geoffrey M. Anderson, Paula Blackstien-Hirsch, Cathy Fooks, and C. David Naylor, eds., *Patterns of Health Care in Ontario*, 2nd ed. (Ottawa: Canadian Medical Association, 1996).

Historical background on the development of health care in Canada may be found in: Wendy Mitchinson and Janice Dickin McGinnis, eds., *Essays in the History of Canadian Medicine* (Toronto: McClelland and Stewart, 1988); C. David Naylor, ed., *Canadian Health Care and the State: A Century of Evolution* (Montreal: McGill-Queen's University Press, 1992); and S.E.D. Shortt, ed., *Medicine in Canadian Society: Historical Perspectives*, first pub. 1981, reprint (Montreal: McGill-Queen's University Press, 1992).

Essential works on both the evaluation and the contemporary functioning of medicare in Canada are Malcolm G. Taylor, *Health Insurance and Canadian Public Policy: The Seven Decisions that Created the Canadian Health Insurance System* (Montreal: McGill-Queen's University Press, 1978), and C. David Naylor, *Private Practice, Public Payment, Canadian Medicine and the Politics of Health Insurance 1911–1966* (Montreal: McGill-Queen's University Press, 1986). Later developments in the relationship between health policy and government are discussed in Joan Price Boase, *Shifting Sands: Government–Group Relationships in the Health Care Sector* (Montreal: McGill-Queen's University Press, 1994). Of particular significance to this volume is a recent study of the sociological characteristics of physicians under Canadian medicare by Bernard Blishen entitled *Doctors in Canada: The Changing World of Medical Practice* (Toronto: University of Toronto Press, 1991).

Two valuable studies by economists are Robert G. Evans, *Strained Mercy: The Economics of Canadian Health Care* (Toronto: Butterworths, 1983), and Malcolm C. Brown, *Health Economics and Policy: Problems and Prescriptions* (Toronto: McClelland and Stewart, 1991).

General works and edited collections on the contemporary Canadian health care system include: David Coburn, Carl D'Arcy, George M. Torrance, and Peter New, eds., *Health and Canadian Society, Sociological Perspectives*, 2nd ed. (Toronto: Fitzhenry and Whiteside, 1987); Anne Crichton, David Hsu, and Stella Tsang, *Canada's Health Care System: Its Funding and Organization*, rev. ed. (Ottawa: Canadian Hospital Association, 1994); Jane Fulton, *Canada's Health Care System: Bordering on the Possible* (New York: Faulkner and Grey, 1993); Raisa B. Deber, and Gail G. Thompson, eds., *Restructuring Canada's Health Services System: How Do We Get There from Here?* (Toronto: University of Toronto Press, 1992); and Ralph W. Sutherland and M. Jane Fulton, *Health Care in Canada: A Description and Analysis of Canadian Health Services*, first pub. 1988, reprint (Ottawa: The Health Group, 1990).

Finally, a number of recent studies have stressed ways of reforming the current system, among which are Doug Angus, Ludwig Auer, J. Eden Cloutier, and Terry Albert, *Sustainable Health for Canada* (Ottawa: Queen's–University of Ottawa Economic Projects, 1995); Pat Armstrong, Hugh Armstrong, Jacqueline Choiniere, Gina Feldberg, and Jerry White, *Take Care: Warning Signals for Canada's Health System* (Toronto: Garamond Press, 1994); Ake Blomqvist and David M. Brown, eds., *Limits to Care: Reforming Canada's Health System in an Age of Restraint* (Toronto: C.D. Howe Institute, 1994); Michael B. Decter, *Healing Medicine, Managing Health System Change the Canadian Way* (Toronto: McGilligan Books, 1994); John L. Dorlan and S. Mathwin Davis, eds., *How Many Roads ... ? Regionalization and Devolution in Heath Care* (Kingston: School of Policy Studies, Queen's University, 1996); Marianne Lamb, Raisa Deber, C. David Naylor, and John E.F. Hastings, *Managed Care in Canada: The Toronto Hospital's Proposed Comprehensive Health Organization* (Ottawa: Canadian Hospital Association Press, 1991); Michael Rachlis and Carol Kushner, *Second Opinion: What's Wrong with Canada's Health-Care System and How to Fix It* (Toronto: Collins, 1989) and *Strong Medicine: How to Save Canada's Health Care System* (Toronto: Harper Collins, 1994); and Ralph Sutherland and Jane Fulton, *Spending Smarter and Spending Less: Policies and Partnerships for Health Care in Canada* (Ottawa: The Health Group, 1994).

Index